By the authors

The Whartons' Stretch Book

The Whartons'

strength
book

The Whartons'
strength
book

Thirty-five Lifts for over
Fifty-five Different Sports and Activities

Jim and Phil Wharton
with Bev Browning

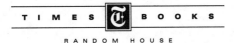
TIMES BOOKS

RANDOM HOUSE

Library of Congress Cataloging-in-Publication Data

Wharton, Jim
    The Whartons' strength book / by Jim and Phil Wharton. — 1st ed.
      p.   cm.
    Includes index.
    ISBN 0-8129-2929-2
    1. Weight training. 2. Bodybuilding. I. Wharton, Phil, 1967– .
II. Title.
GV546W52   1999
613.7'13—dc21   98-19990

Random House website address: www.atrandom.com

Printed in the United States of America
9 8 7 6 5 4 3 2

First Edition

For the athletes, dancers, clients, and
healthcare professionals who share our lives
and our work every day.

Acknowledgments

Thank you so much to Michael Browning, who took us into his family while we worked with Bev to write this book. Many thanks to Reid Boates, the world's greatest agent, and Elizabeth Rapoport, the world's greatest editor. Thanks so much to our colleague and friend, Exercise Physiologist Greg Young, MS, CSCS, who opened his library and shared his experience with us. Thanks for the generous efforts and talents of Shannon Silcox, Ron Boyle, Jill Werman, Randy Brower, Tom Nohilly, Salisha Abraham, Gordon Gow, and Michelle Assaf. Special thanks and love to Hugh Hubbard ("Isn't it grand?"). Thanks to the United States Olympic Committee for their assistance with our section on drugs and supplements. Thanks to the USDA. Thanks to Laura Hallam with the Florida Governor's Council on Physical Fitness and Sports. Thanks to the U.S. National Senior Sports Organization in Washington, DC. Thanks to Shane Powers, the Assistant Manager at Hunters Crossing Publix Supermarket in Gainesville, Florida, who opened his store before hours, and helped us weigh and measure groceries for our section, "Clean and Jerk." Thanks to the strength and conditioning pioneers who elevated our field from science to art, M. Dena Gardiner, Robert E. Shelton, Leonardo Greninger, and Aaron L. Mattes.

And finally, many thanks to friend and teacher, Michael Pollock, PhD, Director of the Center for Exercise Science, and Professor of the Departments of Medicine and Exercise and Sport Sciences at the University of Florida. You will be missed.

J. W.
P. W.

Contents

Occupations   193

Part IV: The Athlete's Life

Introduction

Active-Isolated Strength with Jim and Phil Wharton

It's new. It's revolutionary. It's the answer for every athlete who has ever asked: "What can I do to maximize my performance?"

It's ACTIVE-ISOLATED STRENGTH.

Written by world-renowned athletic trainers Jim and Phil Wharton for their clients, this book is a portable training guide and a companion to *The Whartons' Stretch Book.*

The Whartons step outside the professional sports arenas and Olympic venues to reveal the secrets of unlocking the human body's full athletic potential. Now, for the first time, YOU can benefit from the experience and expertise of personal trainers who have assisted such athletes as Art Monk, Wanda Panfill, Nelson Diebel, Anthony Nesty, Bob Arnot, and Jack Pierce.

Those are just some of their credentials. From here on, the Whartons will tell you themselves about what Active-Isolated Strength can do for you.

ACTIVE-ISOLATED STRENGTH WORK:
THE ATHLETE'S SECRET WEAPON

A few years ago, we stood in a well-known gym and watched as a fitness trainer worked with a client. The man was kneeling under a bar that was suspended on a cable and pulley over his head. The client reached up, grasped the bar, pulled it straight down behind his head until it touched his neck, and then slowly relaxed his arms to return it to its starting position. The trainer shouted encouragement, "Good job! Get those deltoids burning!" The trainer might have been well intentioned, but the deltoids weren't getting much of a workout. From our vantage point, we could see the client's muscles as they fired. We watched as his abdominals, shoulders, arms, neck extensors, hip flexors, quads, hamstrings, and whole back were engaged to assist the pull down and keep him in alignment on his knees. A lot of muscles were involved, but none was getting a good workout. And most certainly not the deltoids.

What went wrong? Nothing actually. The body was doing what it is supposed to do. Mother Nature designed the muscles to be helpful to each other. When one is weak, fatigued, cramped, or struggling, the body automatically recruits volunteers—other muscles that can kick in to get the job done. When the body recruits volunteer muscles to assist a weak and struggling muscle, the weaker muscle gets shut out and stays weak. And the recruited muscles get a . . . sort of . . . workout.

That's the problem. When a person works out using conventional methods, there is no accommodation for this phenomenon.

A slight shift in the focus of the workout could make a big difference. In conventional strength training, we work out to *lift a weight.* What if we slightly shift the focus so that the goal is to *strengthen a weak muscle,* instead of lift a weight?

Active-Isolated Strength methodically isolates muscles, so your body will not be able to recruit. It activates ONLY the targeted area. Using weights and the resistance of your own body when you work out, you activate or "fire" muscles one at a time in a prescribed sequence. This is why we call it Active-Isolated Strength work. As you fire one muscle, the opposite muscle will relax for a good stretch, allowing a greater range of motion and a fuller and more complete workout of the firing muscle's fibers, from one end to the other. Adding weight or a greater number of repetitions to the exercises allows you to control the degree of strength of each muscle or the "sculpting-and-shaping" effects you want. In essence, your own body becomes your gym. It's so easy and so much fun that the excuses go away. And you'll start seeing results that will please you.

You'll never grab a bar, pull down, and think "deltoids" again.

We invite you to join our clients on a quest for ultimate fitness with our no-excuses, no-escape workout program.

Active-Isolated Strength work is for anyone who wants to be a player in life. Our clients range from professional athletes to weekend warriors. We work with people who want to lose fat, rehabilitate from an injury, take up a sport for the first time, regain lost vitality, reshape a sagging waistline, get bigger, get smaller, get fitter. No matter what your motivation is, the benefits and rewards of fitness are impressive. You'll feel, look, sleep, eat, perform, and function better. You'll be healthier. You'll be more alert, and your senses will be heightened. It's an attractive package. It's yours by birthright. All it takes is a little time (less than conventional methods) and effort (less than you might imagine). And Active-Isolated Strength works.

We have a friend—clearly a weekend warrior—- who tells everyone she meets that she is training for the Olympics. When we try from time to time to interject a little reality into her fitness goals, she curtly reminds us that she *can* train for the Olympics if she wants to. She's right. Anyone can.

ANYONE CAN TRAIN FOR THE OLYMPICS

We're serious. You can train with all the gusto of the Olympic spirit, even if (like our friend) you never really intend to show up at the Trials. Olympic-caliber training programs are basic, and the principles are universal and as old as time. Only the applications are new, thanks to state-of-the-art scientific research and emerging biomechanical information. We ought to know. We've been training professional and amateur athletes for years. And we'll tell you something that will shock you. It doesn't take a high-tech gym to train for the Olympics. Athletes from all over the world train, qualify for their national teams, compete, and WIN without ever stepping foot into a fitness center. It's the best-kept secret around. One of our favorite stories is about the famous Finnish Olympic track champion Emil Zatopek, who trained for his three gold medals by putting his wife on his back—piggyback-style—and running up and down the stairs in their home when it was too cold and snowy to train outside. Getting strong is a simple matter of physics in cahoots with biology. You stress a muscle with weight. It resists. It rests. It gets stronger. Easy, right? Well, almost. You have to know which muscles to stress, how, how often, and how long. But don't worry. We're here to help. That's why we wrote this book.

You're about to become fit—and stay that way—with the help of a *personal training program* that maximizes your efforts and minimizes your time expenditure. Quality rather than quantity—and knowing exactly what you're doing, and doing it right—will give you the results and benefits you want.

As trainers with years of experience, we can assure you that Active-Isolated Strength work is very real. Between the covers of this book, you will find workout programs designed for you. These programs are:

- Adaptable to any level of skill, even as you get better and stronger.

- Backed by sound scientific principles and documented research.

- Dependent on no special facilities or equipment.

- Designed for maximum results with efficient, time-saving effort.

- Explained in simple-to-follow instructions.

- Identical to the programs used by many champion Olympic and professional athletes.

- No-cost to low-cost.

- Specifically tailored to your personal goals or your specific sport.

Besides, they're so much fun that you'll have no difficulty in putting strength training into your life, and keeping it there.

FIRST THINGS FIRST

As with any fitness program, you should check with your physician to make certain that you are well enough to enjoy the benefits of working out.

The Seven Myths of Strength Training

The world of strength training is saturated with misinformation passed on from one well-intentioned athlete to another. Since the dawn of lifting, athletes have cornered each other in locker rooms and whispered, "Say, what do YOU think about . . . ?" The person being asked is naturally flattered but is too busy folding his towel at the moment to dash out to medical school for a degree in sports medicine, so he comes up with an answer—likely the same one that *he* got when he asked someone. We call this passing along of information "Aboriginal Coaching." The tradition originates from storytelling around the campfire, where one warrior impresses the others with his vast knowledge about any given subject. The problem in strength training is that myth and wonderment have etched some pretty far-fetched ideas into the theory and practice. It's no one's fault, really. In the very beginning of strength training, there was no research. Everyone just did the best they could. Only since researchers have entered the picture, and athletes have moved from their gyms into gleaming laboratories, have we some concrete science to back up (or debunk) our theories. Frankly, science intervened in the nick of time. With a full-blown fitness revolution taking place, more people are participating in fitness programs than at any other time in history. Unfortunately, it takes a long time to correct long-held, sacred, wrong beliefs. Fitness professionals all over the world are doing their best to make corrections as quickly as possible, to prevent mistakes in training on a grand scale, and to get people on the right track. In our clinic, we say, "What you don't know CAN hurt you, but what you THINK you know can hurt you even worse!" We call these tidbits of misinformation the "Myths of Strength Training." They are so universally accepted that you have probably heard them and may believe some of them to be true. It's time to set the record straight. And we are just the guys to do it! (By the way, if you thought that any of these myths were gospel truth, please don't feel bad about being misinformed. You were in good company. Still, it's best that you don't admit to anyone that you were duped.)

Myth 1. No pain, no gain! Right?

WRONG!   The "No pain, no gain" mantra is the sadistic companion of "Go for the burn!" Every time we hear it, we want to snatch a trainer up by his shorts and beat him with a 1980s fitness video. No wonder people have been avoiding working out! The perception is that unless training hurts, it isn't doing you any good. Having pain tell you that something is right goes against the laws of nature. Pain is Mother Nature's loud, clear signal that your body is being damaged and that you need to stop whatever you're doing. In fact, your brain is programmed to instantaneously react (without your having to think about it) to wrench you away from a pain stimulus. Also, in sports training and rehabilitation, pain is used as a diagnostic tool for pinpointing injury, getting an initial measure of its severity, and comparing subsequent readings on the progress of healing. So pain is a very good thing. We love pain. Many things in life are SUPPOSED to hurt, like running over your own foot with a lawn mower, but working out is not one of them.

We can see you getting ready to issue an objection. After all, you've *seen* runners grimacing down the road and weight lifters screaming and sweating. You think it looks painful. In a sense, you would be right . . . a little. Working out can be uncomfortable and require great effort. It can and does take you to the limit. But actual PAIN is where that limit is. Once you've hit that threshold between "uncomfortable" and "painful," you draw back before you do damage.

Working out is fun. It takes you back to human basics where you'll rediscover joy. You're supposed to have a good time.

Myth 2. You can lose inches off your waist in just weeks with the ab (abdominal conditioning) machine! Right?

WRONG!   Manufacturers' claims have a whole lot of starry-eyed people spending big bucks for roll bars and throwing themselves onto the floor to crunch. If you're one of those people, we wish you had called us first. We could have saved you a bundle and helped you keep your carpet clean. The claim is false on two fronts. First, there's no such thing as spot reducing. Sorry. When you build muscle and burn extra calories, your body decides what fat goes first. You can't crunch your abdomen and demand that only abdominal fat melts off. If you burn calories, they are drawn from all over, in a genetically programmed sequence over which you have no control. And second, you can't get fit in weeks. Well, you *can,* if you put enough of them back to back—perhaps as many as 52.

Here's one final irony that ends the fantasies of many spot-reducers. In attempting to spot-reduce by overexercising one area of your body, you'll likely pump that muscle group up and make it larger. If your goal is to get smaller, this is the last thing you want. (It's rumored that Popeye was only trying to lose a few pesky inches off his forearms!)

Myth 3. Exercising to failure is the best strategy for strengthening a muscle! Right?

WRONG!   Training to failure is repeating a motion until you can't do it anymore. Here's how it works. As you lift, some of your muscles become fatigued and drop out. Theoretically, in the split second after that happens, other muscles are recruited to take up the slack, and you get some pretty sneaky compounded benefit. Not only do the muscles in the primary group get a really good, hard workout, but some secondary muscles are recruited and stressed, even if only momentarily. Sorry to tell you: That's not true. The truth is that no studies have been able to directly examine training to failure versus not training to failure, because it's been impossible for researchers to figure out how to equalize the work in the laboratory. One attempt at quantifying results measured the performance effects of one set to failure, three sets to failure, and a periodized program (no training to failure). All sets were eight to twelve repetitions each. Guess what they found at the end of seven weeks? In all exercises, the people who did not exercise to failure performed equal to or better than those who pumped till they pooped.

The problem with working out to failure is that you damage the muscle. Heavy weight training—especially on large muscles—can lead to overuse injury in an astonishingly short period of time. Before long, the athlete will notice that no gains are being made and, worse, injured muscles are weakening. Additionally, experts cite alarming statistics regarding acute injuries in tendons.

More bad news. Training to fatigue in young athletes damages the growth plates in bones. Also, the highest spike in blood pressure occurs at the moment of failure. If an athlete has hypertension, this could be dangerous.

Myth 4. Searing pain is due to a buildup of lactic acid! Right?

WRONG! Lactic acid in your muscles does burn, but its presence is often described as "discomfort that builds slowly." Lactic acid is only one of the metabolic waste products that your body produces as muscles fire and undergo microtraumas. If your body is unable to keep up with the demand for flushing these waste products out of your muscles, those muscle fibers begin to get irritated and to fatigue. When you work out hard, you rapidly become familiar with the sensations of buildup, and use them to monitor your exertion levels and make decisions regarding performance: pour it on, or back it off. Searing pain is very different. It's an indicator that something has been suddenly and traumatically injured. You might have a strain, a sprain, a nerve impingement, a tear, or a fracture; lactic acid is the least of your problems. Stop whatever you're doing IMMEDIATELY (unless you're dialing 911).

Myth 5. If I stop working out, my muscles will turn to fat! Right?

WRONG! Not unless you are an alchemist or a genetic mutant. Here's a basic anatomy lesson: "Muscle is muscle and fat is fat." You can't turn one into the other. (If we could, we would work the other way, wave our magic Wharton wands, and turn fat into muscle!) What really happens when an athlete stops working out is that his or her caloric demand decreases dramatically. In a later chapter (page 209), we explain that one of the secret and wicked delights of athletes is that we can eat daily caloric intakes that would shock the celery-nibblers (if we told them). Not only is eating perfectly all right, but it's necessary to fuel the performance efforts we demand from our bodies. Remember, "Food is fuel" and athletes need full tanks of high-test. The problem with abandoning the activity that made all this necessary is that the body no longer requires as many calories. Unfortunately, it's difficult to adjust eating habits to accommodate this diminished need. Often, it's not the athlete's fault. It's a fine balancing act, as difficult to achieve as figuring out how to keep from losing weight when your intake is 6,000 calories a day.

One more insidious thing happens. After only 72 hours have passed since the last workout, the body begins a gentle, almost undetectable slide into sloth. In time, muscle mass diminishes. Finely tuned muscles that used to fire, burn calories, and juice up metabolism just can't do the job anymore. Consequently, the body does not burn fat particularly efficiently. So the fat gain accelerates, compounded by a declining metabolism, diminishing muscle mass, and failure to adjust caloric intake. Muscle does NOT turn into fat. The fat just takes over. The trick, of course, is to continue working out at some level.

Myth 6. **Sweat suits and wide neoprene waist cinchers melt inches and pounds away while I lift! Right?**

WRONG! Your body turns up the heat when you work out. Your muscles are like little furnaces, thermodynamically converting calories into energy to fuel your effort. You need more oxygen for this internal ignition process, so your heart beats faster and you breathe harder. Your whole system revs up. And you get hot. As that happens, your body has to maintain your core temperature to keep your internal organs cool, so it generates sweat that evaporates off your skin and naturally cools you off. The whole process is a miracle in efficiency . . . and all engineered by Mother Nature to save your spleen from being parboiled. Now, if you swaddle yourself in a sweat suit—or worse, a neoprene body stocking—you interfere with the Grand Design. You generate more heat, which in turn generates more sweat. And, as if you haven't done enough, you block your body's ability to take advantage of evaporation and cool its core—*your vital organs,* including what's left of your brain. As for limiting the neoprene to a belt, we've already told you that spot-reducing is impossible, so although wearing a belt wouldn't be as bad as covering your entire body, it would be useless.

We'll admit that, if you make yourself sweat, you WILL lose weight. But the weight you lose will be water. Sweat; you'll end up dehydrated. Your workout will be trashed. You'll gain back all your weight loss at the water fountain, but you're going to stay in a dehydrated state for up to 48 hours, while your cells recover their volume. What you really want to do is lose FAT, not weight. Weight is irrelevant; it's an ever-changing number that reflects the composition of your entire body: water, bone, tissue, muscle, fat, hair, and sneakers. It makes a lot more sense to give your body every opportunity to get a good workout. It can then rev up its metabolic furnaces and get stronger, so you can burn more calories and get leaner. Be cool. Literally.

Myth 7. If I work out, I'll bulk up! Right?

WRONG! While many people do train to build muscle mass and bulk up, bulking up isn't the inevitable outcome of strength work. In fact, you'll have to engage in very specific workout protocols—heavy weights and repeated sets—to do it. Getting stronger without enlarging your muscles is as simple as lifting lighter weights with more repetitions and limited sets. If you aren't interested in bulking up, exercise physiologists and researchers tell us that a more "conservative" development can give you just as much strength as a pumped-up, bulging form. In fact, the size of a muscle is not an accurate measure of its strength. In any effort to sculpt a body, bigger is not necessarily better. In fact, studies suggest that the larger development puts extra weight and demand on the body, and may impede the ability to move a muscle through its full range of motion—creating, ironically, weakness in some of the muscle's function.

We most often hear this concern over bulking up from women, who want to get leaner and stronger but still maintain soft curves. Working out will not turn you into the Hulk . . . unless you want it to. (And, again, you're going to have to put major effort into this.) Unlike your male counterparts at the gym, your body is lined with a subcutaneous layer of fat. Mother Nature put it there to insulate unborn children and to store estrogen. It's entirely possible for you to be highly developed muscularly, and yet keep that physique "hidden" and create a soft line. Instead of appearing to be "ripped" and "cut"—which you may very well be—you'll maintain a smoother topography. To show detailed muscular development, you would have to reduce the layer of fat to levels well below normal for females. Keep in mind that male body builders display definition by lowering their fat content to below 4 percent. If this seems like a good plan for women, forget it. Dropping your fat content below 16 percent may cause your estrogen levels to diminish, possibly resulting in your losing estrogen's cardioprotective properties, developing amenorrhea, and running an increased risk of osteoporosis. Every woman is different, so you and your physician will want to monitor your body carefully and make intelligent decisions that take into consideration the long-term consequences of dieting into low ranges of body fat.

Strong, fit, healthy women are beautiful women . . . soft curves included.

Can a woman bulk up? You bet. But be advised that you will never be as massive as your male counterparts. You just aren't genetically programmed to achieve that physique. Male lifters have the benefit of testosterone, which facilitates muscle building. While it's true that you have a measure of testosterone in your system, too, you simply do not have as much as men do. You might have heard that you can remedy this by taking supplements, but we forbid you to be this stupid. Not only could you ruin your health, destroy your ability to have children, and shorten your "bulked up" life, but you will probably also grow facial hair, break out in widespread acne, deepen your voice, become aggressive, get depressed, and develop unnatural urges to urinate standing up and to hunt for your own food. We insist that you seek to develop your body only to the extent that you are genetically permitted. You'll enjoy the results.

Part I

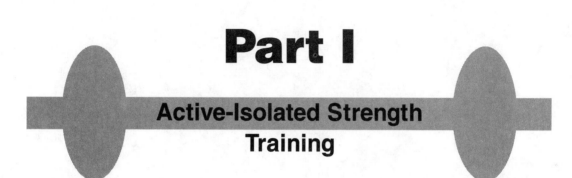

Active-Isolated Strength Training

Notes for Athletes

We work with athletes every day, and we know one immutable truth about you. Your body is a miracle. Not only is your body astonishing in its complexity and efficiency, but it works hard—through a series of valiant compensations—to overcome every abuse and any neglect it suffers. Throughout your lifetime, it constantly tries to bring itself back to perfect function and form. When it's injured, your body rallies to heal. Where there is imbalance, it adjusts to counterbalance. When you limit your caloric intake, it lowers your metabolism. Where your body has a weakness, it recruits other muscles to get its job done. Your body is designed to get it right. Toward that end, it responds dramatically to training. That's the good news. The great news is that it's never too late to put exercise into your life or to fine-tune an already good training program.

Recently, we were discussing physiological and psychological strategies for running the punishing 26.2 miles of a marathon, specifically after that notorious twentieth mile, when fatigue sets in and one's thinking becomes a little vague. (This is a nice way to say, "You've bonked!") We all agreed that the marathon is a strategic race. The runner must *think* his or her way through the course, setting up a sort of master command center in the brain from which decisions and adjustments can be made regarding such matters as stride, pacing, body carriage, route, focus, hydration, nutrition, and pain. But what happens when fatigue causes confusion and crossed signals in the master command center? Phil says his body just takes over. It *knows* what to do. His muscles are trained and imprinted with "knowledge" on a cellular level. And his instincts are already set on "cruise control" to finish the race. At that moment in the marathon, when his ability to think and make decisions is (ever so slightly!) impaired, Phil trusts his body completely. They're partners and know each other well enough to know the job will get done. It's an interesting way to look at the mind–body connection.

The partnership between an athlete and his or her body comes from experience and knowledge. Training is always more effective if you understand how the body works, so settle back for a basic anatomy lesson as we introduce you to the wonders and miracles under your clothes.

AN OBSCENELY SHORT VERSION OF ANATOMY 101

Of all the tissues in your body, by far the majority—some 40 percent of your total mass—is muscle. Simply put, muscles' jobs are to move you and to "brake" you to stop you from moving. Muscles are neatly packaged in sheaths or capsules to help them hold their shapes, retain their lubricants, and keep them from sticking to each other. They are organized and attached to a rigid frame—approximately 206 bones in your skeleton—either directly or by tendons. Those 206 bones are attached to each other by superbly engineered interlocking systems called ligaments. Where two bones adjoin but need to move (such as in your knee), the two ends of the bones will be covered with a smooth elastic covering called cartilage, which provides a frictionless joint and absorbs shock. Muscles are fired—contracted to move—by signals from the brain that are transmitted through the nerves. Blood flow brings nutrients and oxygen to muscles, and carries away their waste. Organs such as the brain, liver, lungs, stomach, and intestines have specific functions to keep everything working and balanced. And skin keeps it all from spilling out onto the ground. Basically, that's your anatomy.

Now that you have the general idea, let's go into some real detail and apply that information to training principles that will help you get stronger faster.

The first step to any good training program is to make the decision that you are going to do a better job at getting fit. Tell yourself:

1. You'll be better able to predict the results of your workouts.

2. You'll have more control over your training processes.

3. You'll achieve efficient results in minimum time.

MAJOR POSTERIOR MUSCLES

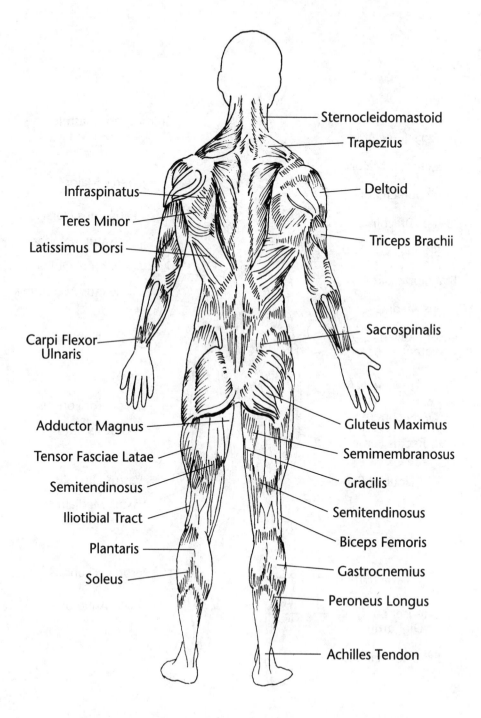

Sternocleidomastoid

Trapezius

Deltoid

Infraspinatus

Teres Minor

Triceps Brachii

Latissimus Dorsi

Carpi Flexor
Ulnaris

Sacrospinalis

Adductor Magnus

Tensor Fasciae Latae

Semitendinosus

Iliotibial Tract

Plantaris

Soleus

Gluteus Maximus

Semimembranosus

Gracilis

Semitendinosus

Biceps Femoris

Gastrocnemius

Peroneus Longus

Achilles Tendon

MAJOR ANTERIOR MUSCLES

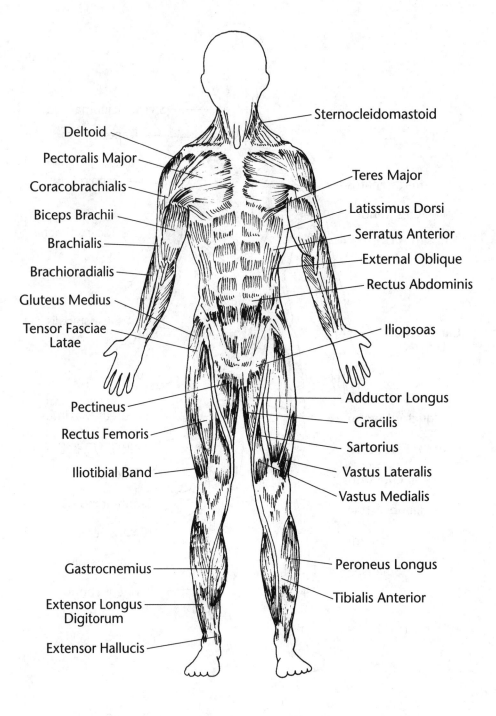

Deltoid

Pectoralis Major

Coracobrachialis

Biceps Brachii

Brachialis

Brachioradialis

Gluteus Medius

Tensor Fasciae Latae

Pectineus

Rectus Femoris

Iliotibial Band

Gastrocnemius

Extensor Longus Digitorum

Extensor Hallucis

Sternocleidomastoid

Teres Major

Latissimus Dorsi

Serratus Anterior

External Oblique

Rectus Abdominis

Iliopsoas

Adductor Longus

Gracilis

Sartorius

Vastus Lateralis

Vastus Medialis

Peroneus Longus

Tibialis Anterior

DESIGNING YOUR ACTIVE-ISOLATED STRENGTH WORKOUT—PUTTING THE PIECES TOGETHER

This book is a training guide and a catalog. Take a few minutes to get comfortable with how to use it.

The rest of this Part I gives you tips, cautions, terminology, advice on clothing and equipment, and some encouragement about your goals. Don't skip any of it. You'll need it all. Schedules for long and short workout programs, and a sample log for your workouts, can be copied and adapted to your personal needs and available time.

Part II catalogs thirty-five specific exercises. They are numbered for your reference throughout the book. The list has been organized to coordinate with five body Zones, as follows:

Zone	Workout Regions	Exercises
1	Upper Legs, Hips, and Trunk	1–15
2	Shoulders	16–25
3	Neck	26
4	Arms, Elbows, Wrists, and Hands	27–30
5	Lower Legs, Ankles, and Feet	31–35

When you select your sports and/or occupations in Part III, you'll have a handy guide for your workouts. Often, all five Zones are listed, but some activities may concentrate on only three or four Zones. That information always precedes the Coaches' Notes in Part III.

Part IV will school you gently and entertainingly in the role of an athlete. Diet, performance, incentives, and rewards are all important. Reinforce your hard work and determination with a new and satisfying self-image. You will have earned it!

THE BASICS OF DESIGNING YOUR PROGRAM

Before you begin designing your personal Active-Isolated Strength program, decide what you want to accomplish. Perhaps you want to slim down and tone up. Perhaps you want to train for a specific sport or activity. Perhaps you want to sculpt and bulk up. Active-Isolated Strength makes each goal possible. Customizing the program to suit you is a simple matter of modifying the routine to give you the workouts you need to get a specific job done. There are three variables you can modify:

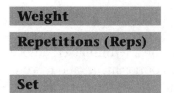

Weight **The weight of the object you lift.**

Repetitions (Reps) **How many times you lift the object after you pick it up.**

Set **A specified series of reps that begins when you pick the weight up for the first time and ends when you put it down for the last time.**

THE WHARTON "BAM"

When we're looking at an overview of a good general-base strengthening program, we see it in three distinct phases. We call it BAMMING an athlete:

B: Building muscular strength (at least a month to get started).

A: Attaining proficiency and musculoskeletal balance (at least six months, although you'll see results more quickly).

M: Maintaining structural integrity (for life).

Although there are no hard-and-fast time lines, you'll know when you move from one phase to the next. The first phase is an adaptation phase: your body adjusts to the increasing demands, and you develop discipline and get used to your equipment. Although the gains you make are significant, they're not as finely tuned as they will be in the second phase. During the attaining phase, you really begin to achieve the results you're after. You adjust each lift until you find power, strength, and balance to give yourself the body you want. You'll stay in this phase until you've discovered that "perfect" place, where everything works just right. In the final phase, maintenance, you'll adjust your workouts to hold on to the fitness you've achieved. This is the easiest of the three phases. Once you've hit it, you might even find yourself able to ease the intensity and frequency of your workouts (although we bet you'll love working out so much that you won't want to).

TO SLIM DOWN AND TONE UP

Light weights.
Eight to twelve reps.
One set.

How much weight is "light" for you? Select a weight you can easily handle. Start with 3 to 5 pounds and see how that feels. Lift the weight for 8 to 12 reps. If the last lift takes no effort, then the weight is too light. You need to increase the increment of the weight slowly until you find your magic number. When you feel mild exertion on the twelfth rep, you've got the right weight to begin. Don't think you can make up for light weight with increased reps or more sets. If the weight is too light, you can lift it forever and all you'll do is burn a few calories. Another thing to remember is that you're stronger in some muscles than in others. One weight might not be sufficient for your purposes. For example, your quadriceps might be more powerful than your wrists. So you might want to purchase or make (see below) a few different weights.

TO SCULPT AND BULK UP

Heavy weights.
Five to eight reps.
One to two sets.

How much weight is "heavy" for you? Select a weight that requires a small amount of effort to lift on the first rep. Lift it for five to eight reps. If the last rep gets your attention, puts a furrow in your brow, and threatens to momentarily break you into a tiny sweat, then you have a weight that is "heavy." If you can't lift through the eighth rep, the weight is too heavy. After you've rested the muscle, decrease the amount of weight by a couple of pounds and try again.

MANAGING A WEIGHT

After you've selected your base weight—the one you'll start with—and worked out with it for a while, it won't take long before it's too light. You'll know it's time to step up the weight when you complete the last rep of the last set without exertion. Increase the weight in small amounts—no more than a pound or two at a time. When you increase the weight, back off a couple of reps until you adjust to the new increment. Remember that increasing the weight for one lift doesn't mean you can automatically increase the weight for all of them.

Managing a weight doesn't always mean finding ways of increasing it. There will come a day when you simply can't lift as much weight as you did the day before. Don't be alarmed. This is just an "off" day. Everyone has them. Back off the weight, reps, or sets until you can manage the workout. Or skip the workout, get some rest, and try again tomorrow. If you don't recover quickly or you notice a consistent decline in your ability to lift, see a physician.

MANAGING A REP

A rep is a smooth lift, generally in two phases. First, you flex or contract the muscle; then you extend or elongate it. A simple way to think about a rep is "Pick it up, put it down" or "Pull it in, push it out." Each exercise in Part II has specific instructions. Your movement should be slow and consistent. Warning! If you like to energize your workout with music that has a fast-paced tempo, you'll have to resist the urge to lift in time to each beat of the music. Move with alternate beats, or at the start of a new measure or line. Exhale slowly as you contract for 2 to 3 seconds. Nice and easy. This gives your muscle time to recruit most of its fibers into the lift. Take the lift all the way to the fullest contraction you can. Hold. Then inhale as you extend the muscle for 3 to 4 seconds. Still nice and easy. Take the extension all the way to the greatest elongation you can. Don't cut it short. Hold. And then flow into the next contraction for the beginning of the next rep. Control the lift completely without swinging the weight up or dropping it down. The lift should be difficult, but not killer. We don't subscribe to "lift to failure"—the practice of lifting until the athlete is unable to manage one more rep. We can't find any literature or research that indicates that this practice is any more effective than lifting until it's difficult. And frankly, cumulative fatigue, which will trash a later workout and carries the possibility of injury, creates more risk than we're willing to take with any of our athletes. You included.

MANAGING SETS

There are two ways to manage your sets. The first is to do all the sets from one lift consecutively on the same muscle or muscle group before you move to the next lift. In other words, if you're doing three sets of each lift, you might do ten reps of quadriceps work, rest, do ten more reps, rest, and do ten more reps before you move on to the next lift. The second way to manage a set is called "Circuit Training": doing one set of everything and then starting all over again. You might find this particularly useful if you work out in a fitness center and you're sensitive about clogging up the flow of clients by doing ten sets per piece of equipment. Circuit Training allows you to move quickly through the line of machines and then take your place in line to begin again. In spite of our concern for your popularity rating at the gym (we would hate to see you get stuffed into your locker), we recommend that you complete all the sets for one lift at one time. The workout is more efficient.

Research in human performance conclusively demonstrates that each set after the first one delivers only an 11 percent gain in benefit. The second and third sets are worth the effort, but make that first one really count: high intensity and technical perfection.

A WORD ABOUT TRAINING FOR A SPECIFIC SPORT

In Part III, Coaches' Notes, each activity is accompanied by suggestions and exercises that we've specifically selected either to give you supplemental strength for the activity or to make up for all the work that the activity will never provide. There is no question that strength training is a vital component in building a fit and healthy athlete. But the bad news is that strength training isn't enough. Nothing you will ever do in the gym will substitute for the activity itself. Researchers who have studied athletes exhaustively have proven that there are factors in activity that are far too complex and elegant to be replicated in the lab (or the gym). If you're going to be a good runner, you have to run. If you're going to be a good tennis player, you have to play tennis. If you're going to be a good oarsman, you have to row. The sport itself is the "sport-specific" workout you're looking for. If you can't participate in your sport for a given period of time, it's possible to simulate some of the neuromuscular patterns of the activity as you work out, but when you return to the playing field—even if you're in the best shape of your life—you'll notice that you're "off" your game. The ability to participate or compete is a tapestry woven with strength, power, finesse, speed, balance, coordination, instinct, reflex, flexibility, endurance, drive, focus, and knowledge. Strength training is an important thread in the tapestry—indeed, it has been called the foundation of all other fitness components. But it's only one thread. Strength training isn't an end; it's a means. Participating in your activities is both. It's the reason you train and it's the way you train. Go have fun!

HOW TO SCHEDULE YOUR ACTIVE-ISOLATED STRENGTH WORKOUT

If you have limited time, the Active-Isolated Strength Short Program is designed for workouts on Monday, Wednesday, and Friday. After you select your activities in Part III, Coaches' Notes, you'll know which exercises to do. Simply put them together on those three days. We would love it if you could sneak in one short abdominal workout EVERY day. And, as your fitness level increases, we encourage you to get more active between workouts, to boost the benefits of your workouts and give you a chance to enjoy your newfound fitness. By the way, you'll notice that Sunday is a day of rest in both the long and short programs. It is intended to be a day when you go out and show off.

    If you have a lot of time, and if you're a serious athlete who is committed to working out every day and can find the time to do it, feel free. In the weekly Workout Log on page 14, we have organized a pattern of workouts that allows rest between sessions that stress one particular muscle group. And, of course, we've sneaked in an abdominal workout (ABS) every day. Please take Sunday off to get good rest and let your body play.

The Active-Isolated Strength Schedules

SHORT PROGRAM

SUNDAY	MONDAY	TUESDAY	WEDNESDAY	THURSDAY	FRIDAY	SATURDAY
Strut Your Stuff!	**All Zones** indicated by your Coaches' Notes		**All Zones** indicated by your Coaches' Notes		**All Zones** indicated by your Coaches' Notes	

LONG PROGRAM

SUNDAY	MONDAY	TUESDAY	WEDNESDAY	THURSDAY	FRIDAY	SATURDAY
Strut Your Stuff!	**ZONE 1** Upper Legs, Hips, and Trunk **ZONE 4** Arms, Elbows, Wrists, and Hands	**DO YOUR ABS!** **ZONE 2** Shoulders **ZONE 3** Neck **ZONE 5** Lower Legs, Ankles, and Feet	**ZONE 1** Upper Legs, Hips, and Trunk **ZONE 4** Arms, Elbows, Wrists, and Hands	**DO YOUR ABS!** **ZONE 2** Shoulders **ZONE 3** Neck **ZONE 5** Lower Legs, Ankles, and Feet	**ZONE 1** Upper Legs, Hips, and Trunk **ZONE 4** Arms, Elbows, Wrists, and Hands	**DO YOUR ABS!** **ZONE 2** Shoulders **ZONE 3** Neck **ZONE 5** Lower Legs, Ankles, and Feet

WHAT TO WEAR

You should always work out in comfortable clothing that allows you to move freely and keeps you cool. We suggest shorts and a T-shirt. Wear nonskid shoes or go barefoot.

WHAT TO BRING TO YOUR WORKOUT

We like to have water and a towel handy, and music is a big favorite in our gym. Scientific studies tell us that you'll get a better workout if you listen to music you like—music with an energetic beat. Also, you might enjoy a large mirror so that you can monitor your form . . . and admire your results.

The Active-Isolated Strength Workout Log

For the Week of _____

SUNDAY	MONDAY	TUESDAY	WEDNESDAY	THURSDAY	FRIDAY	SATURDAY
	PROGRAM	PROGRAM	PROGRAM	PROGRAM	PROGRAM	PROGRAM
	❏ ABS	❏ ABS	❏ ABS	❏ ABS	❏ ABS	❏ ABS
	❏ ZONE 1 Upper Legs, Hips, and Trunk	❏ ZONE 1 Upper Legs, Hips, and Trunk	❏ ZONE 1 Upper Legs, Hips, and Trunk	❏ ZONE 1 Upper Legs, Hips, and Trunk	❏ ZONE 1 Upper Legs, Hips, and Trunk	❏ ZONE 1 Upper Legs, Hips, and Trunk
	❏ ZONE 2 Shoulders	❏ ZONE 2 Shoulders	❏ ZONE 2 Shoulders	❏ ZONE 2 Shoulders	❏ ZONE 2 Shoulders	❏ ZONE 2 Shoulders
	❏ ZONE 3 Neck	❏ ZONE 3 Neck	❏ ZONE 3 Neck	❏ ZONE 3 Neck	❏ ZONE 3 Neck	❏ ZONE 3 Neck
	❏ ZONE 4 Arms, Elbows, Wrists, and Hands	❏ ZONE 4 Arms, Elbows, Wrists, and Hands	❏ ZONE 4 Arms, Elbows, Wrists, and Hands	❏ ZONE 4 Arms, Elbows, Wrists, and Hands	❏ ZONE 4 Arms, Elbows, Wrists, and Hands	❏ ZONE 4 Arms, Elbows, Wrists, and Hands
	❏ ZONE 5 Lower Legs, Ankles, and Feet	❏ ZONE 5 Lower Legs, Ankles, and Feet	❏ ZONE 5 Lower Legs, Ankles, and Feet	❏ ZONE 5 Lower Legs, Ankles, and Feet	❏ ZONE 5 Lower Legs, Ankles, and Feet	❏ ZONE 5 Lower Legs, Ankles, and Feet
	NOTES	NOTES	NOTES	NOTES	NOTES	NOTES
	❏ Drank Plenty of Water	❏ Drank Plenty of Water	❏ Drank Plenty of Water	❏ Drank Plenty of Water	❏ Drank Plenty of Water	❏ Drank Plenty of Water

TIPS FOR SUCCEEDING

1. Keep a weekly record of your workouts. Make photocopies of the Workout Log (p. 14) for your personal use. In the upper box, check the appropriate programs for quick reference. You can do this in advance, so that your workouts are organized weekly. The middle box is for your personal notes, such as "I added an extra set in here" or "I had to quit early" or "Did extra ABS." And the little box at the bottom is a gentle reminder that you need to hydrate. Drinking plenty of fluids is essential to a good workout.

2. Follow the specific order. It's important that you follow the sequence of exercises and do them in the order given. Start each exercise with a warm-up. Go through the motions a few times without weight. This is called a pre-set. It prepares your muscles to work. Work the Zones from 1 to 5, and perform the exercises within the individual Zones in order as well. The workouts are specifically organized to warm up muscles gradually and engage them when they're ready to fire. Don't skip around.

3. Know when you're working out hard enough. If you work out too hard, you'll get exhausted, discouraged, and injured. If you don't work out hard enough, you'll fail to see results and abandon the workout. One of the easiest ways to gauge the level of your intensity is with a **rate of perceived exertion (RPE).** Very simply, you gauge your intensity by asking a basic question: "How do I FEEL?" Sitting stock still in an easy chair will have a rating of 0. Walking at a brisk pace, where you can still talk and haven't thought of throwing up yet, is a 3. Doing something really strenuous, like pushing your car up a hill, is a 9 or 10. For Active-Isolated Strength training, you want to be working out at an RPE between 3 and 5.

4. Keep track of where you are on the RPE Scale.

0   No exertion

1   Very weak

2   Weak

3   Moderate

4   Somewhat strong

5   Strong

6   Stronger

7   Very strong

8   Very, very strong
9   Extremely strong
10   Maximum exertion, uncomfortable

WHEN TOO MUCH OF A GOOD THING IS BAD

Working out is supposed to be fun, but let's be honest. It can be a little uncomfortable, especially when you're working hard. You'll notice that we characterize the sensation of exertion as "uncomfortable," not "painful." This is an important distinction. As you grow more familiar with working out, you'll learn to listen to your "body language" and make decisions based on that information. Until then, here's a vocabulary list of the signals that your body might communicate to alert you that you are pushing too hard, that something's wrong, and that you need to back off.

Pain

At no time should an exercise hurt. Pain is your body's way of identifying a point of injury and, automatically and instantaneously, activating your entire system to wrench you away from whatever is causing injury and protect you from further harm. If you allow an exercise to hurt, you're going to have to override your body's natural instincts to protect itself. That's not easy. Your muscles tighten when they get ready to take flight but are not allowed to flee. Working out a specific muscle when all those around it are firing to deal with pain makes the workout ineffective. More important, it's not smart. Your body is trying to tell you something. Pain is injury. Back off. Rest. Lift lighter weights. Adjust your position. Or quit.

Shortness of Breath

When you exert yourself, your muscles require more oxygen as they fire. So your heart rate goes up and you pant to keep up with demand for air intake. It's part of Mother Nature's grand design for quickly circulating oxygen-rich blood throughout your system when it needs it. However, if you find yourself short of breath—panting without exertion, or unable to breathe deeply or quickly enough to satisfy your body's signals that you need more air—then something is very wrong. Stop the workout immediately, and sit down. If you are unable to recover within a few minutes, dial 911.

Feeling Light-Headed

If you can't take in enough oxygen to meet the demands of your muscles, one of the first organs to experience the deficit is your brain. The symptoms are described as being "light headed" or "feeling faint." A number of things can cause an athlete to feel light-headed: low blood pressure, low blood sugar, fatigue, hunger, medications, shock, illness, overexertion, and cardiovascular or neurological diseases. Stop the workout immediately. You've got two problems. One, of course, is the source of the symptom. The other (and more immediate) one is that, if you faint, you're liable to injure yourself seriously in the fall. Get low immediately. Sit in a chair and put your head between your knees, or lie on the floor and elevate your feet. You should feel better immediately. If not, call for help or, if you're alone and able to get to a phone, dial 911.

Dizziness

Feeling dizzy is similar to feeling light-headed. The causes can be the same, but the symptoms are slightly different. Dizziness takes light-headedness one step further. Your equilibrium and coordination are disturbed. You're unable to focus your eyes on a world that swims around you. Close your eyes and get down on the floor immediately. (Don't try to sit in a chair and put your head between your knees. When you lean forward, you might keep going.) If you can, elevate your feet and call for help. Breathe slowly and deeply. Relax. You should feel better immediately. Test yourself by slowly opening your eyes and affixing your attention on something stationary. If you can focus, try sitting up. Don't get up until you're sure your equilibrium and coordination are back to 100 percent. If you don't feel better, call for help. If you're alone and able to get to a phone, dial 911.

Chest Pain

Chest pain isn't always a heart attack, but it's best to assume the worst, so you can get the best and fastest treatment . . . just in case. Experiencing chest pain while you're working out is serious, no matter what the source. Experts say that all people should know the warning signs of a heart attack because the sooner you get treatment, the less damage your heart will suffer. Look for:

- Sudden, intense pressure or pain in the chest.

- Chest pain that travels to the arm, neck, shoulder, or back.

- Chest discomfort accompanied by light-headedness, fainting, shortness of breath, weakness, nausea, and/or vomiting or sweating.

If these symptoms last more than five minutes—or you have severe heartburn that isn't relieved by antacids—dial 911. While you're waiting for the ambulance to arrive, take an aspirin, lie down, and breathe slowly, all of which may help to limit the damage to your heart muscle.

Shakiness or Trembling

When a muscle is fatigued or damaged, or when the neurological pathway between the brain and the muscle is disrupted, the muscle responds to the brain's call for action with a series of minute contractions or spasms. Instead of firing strongly, it quivers. It's the best it can do. Trembling is common after an unusually hard workout, when an athlete has exerted extraordinary effort. When you feel a specific muscle shaking or trembling, back off and give it a chance to rest. When metabolic waste products clear and the muscle is recovered, likely you'll be fine. If a twenty-four-hour layoff seems to make no difference, see a physician. If you feel shaky in general, stop the workout. Rest and drink plenty of fluids. You're probably just tired, but if you don't feel better in a few hours, see a physician. If the symptoms escalate into light-headedness, feeling faint, shortness of breath, weakness, nausea, or sweating, dial 911.

Throbbing Head

Headaches induced by lifting or gripping might be symptoms of high blood pressure. Although the headache is unpleasant, it's a gift. It's warning you that you might have a big problem—high blood pressure that could lead to stroke. Stop the workout immediately. Rest and drink plenty of fluids. When you feel a little better, hop in your car, get yourself to your physician, and ask for a blood pressure check.

Fatigue

Being tired is part of being human. Learning to tell the difference between being tired and being dangerously tired is part of being an athlete. It's a fine line. Sometimes, when you're tired, working out will energize you. And in the long term, having a healthy, fit body will help give you the stamina you need to beat fatigue that would sideline "mere mortals." On the other hand, if you work out when you're tired, you run the risk of an injury or an ineffective workout, and you're failing to acknowledge the possibly dangerous source of the fatigue. Experience will teach you when to cave in to fatigue and when to leap into a workout in spite of it. We always make that decision based on this questionnaire:

If you answer YES to any of these questions, bag the workout. Take care of the problem, and get back to working out as soon as you're 100 percent.

- Am I tired because I am insufficiently recovered from my last workout?
- Am I ill?
- Has this fatigue gone on longer than a couple of days?
- Am I experiencing any other symptoms besides fatigue?
- Is my resting pulse rate accelerated?
- Am I dehydrated?

If you answer YES to any of the questions below, you can begin the workout. But be extra careful. Avoid sloppy technique or shortcuts that come with being tired. Stick with your program for at least ten minutes. If you don't feel better, bag the workout. Try again tomorrow.

- Am I tired because I had a tough day?
- Did I get enough sleep last night?
- Did I eat well today?
- Does this fatigue have anything to do with my attitude or state of mind?
- Have I been tired like this before, but worked out anyway and felt better?
- Am I just looking for excuses, because I don't feel like working out?

Any Sensation That's Unusual

We all feel things differently and we all have different ways of expressing what we feel. For you to be experiencing any of the above, the vocabulary doesn't have to match exactly. In fact, you might not even be able to describe what you feel, especially if the sensation is new and unfamiliar. Our best advice to you is that if you "feel odd," pay attention and take it seriously. If a symptom or sensation alarms you, or if your instincts tell you that something's wrong, stop the workout immediately and consult a physician. To quote the old cliché, "It's better to be safe than sorry."

IS THERE A "BETTER" TIME OF DAY TO WORK OUT?

Definitely: whenever you can. Some athletes enjoy working out first thing in the morning, to get their bodies moving and awake. This gets the workout out of the way before "life" broadsides a busy schedule. (However, you must promise not to show up for work so pleased with yourself that you become smug and obnoxious in the eyes of your coworkers who couldn't even get their hair combed.) On the other hand, some people feel too sluggish in the morning to get anything moving. They can barely manage to lift a coffee cup, and are just glad if they can knock it over and lap the coffee up off the kitchen table. In their defense, some studies suggest that leaping out of bed and throwing oneself into immediate exertion might put strain on a body that's not warmed up and a heart that's not ready to pound yet. Many people enjoy working out at the end of the day, to release stress and tension. And, contrary to conventional wisdom, working out right before bedtime is not necessarily the dreaded insomnia-producer that we once thought. We do it all the time. (A great surprise benefit of working out—at any time—is that you tire your body physically, so your sleep will improve.)

WHAT IF YOU HAVE TO MISS A WORKOUT?

You'll live. Just get back on your schedule as soon as possible. We'll tell you a little secret. Researchers have clearly demonstrated that it isn't necessary to cram a whole workout into one time slot. If you have to break it up into a lot of little stolen moments, the benefits will be almost as good. If you do this with your Active-Isolated Strength training, remember that the exercises are arranged in a specific order so that muscles are not engaged until they're warmed up and ready. If you leap in and out of the workout, you run the risk of straining something. However, if you keep it light—just for the sake of moving—you'll be all right. Perhaps, instead of Active-Isolated Strength training, you could walk briskly up and down the hall for a few minutes, to get things moving and circulate some blood. Doing something is better than doing nothing—as long as you don't get hurt.

YOU'LL NEED TO GATHER SOME EQUIPMENT

It's time to set up a personal gym. While it's possible to get fit without equipment, it's a whole lot easier and faster if you work out with weights. At the beginning of each exercise, we tell you what you'll need. Quickly review the lists below, and compile a little collection of your own.

If you're on a sky's-the-limit budget, purchase:

2 5-pound ankle weights.

2 2.5-pound ankle weights.

2 10-pound ankle weights.

2 5-pound dumbbells.

1 8-foot length of thick nylon rope.

1 dowel.

1 rope.

1 pair of tube socks.

1 full-size bath towel.

If you're on a somewhat limited budget, purchase:

2 5-pound ankle weights.

1 5-pound dumbbell.

1 8-foot length of thick nylon rope.

1 pair of tube socks.

1 full-size bath towel.

If you're on an extremely limited budget, purchase:

1 5-pound ankle weight.

1 5-pound dumbbell.

1 8-foot length of thick nylon rope.
   (You can borrow the belt from your bathrobe, or tie a couple of leather belts together, or take down your clothesline.)

1 pair of tube socks.
   (Look down. You're wearing them. Take one off and you're all set.)

1 full-size bath towel.
   (Walk into the bathroom and get yourself a towel. Just make sure it's not in use at the time.)

EQUIPMENT UNDER YOUR NOSE

We promised you that this was a "no-excuses" workout program and we meant it. If rain nor sleet nor snow nor dark of night will deter us from getting fit, then mere money (or lack of it) will not stand in our way! If you don't want to spend very much money, or if you find yourself on the road without your workout equipment, don't despair or skip a workout. Necessity is the mother of invention, and more than one athlete has improvised his or her way to fitness. Milo of Crotana, the six-time Olympic Games champion in the sixth century B.C., lifted a growing calf on his shoulders every day until it was fully grown, and may very well have invented progressive strength training as we know it today. Even without access to actual livestock, we have constructed entire gyms out of things we found in hotel rooms and grocery stores. It's really pretty simple. All you need to do is determine how much weight you need, and then find something that weighs that much and is safe to lift.

A LAUNDRY LIST OF WEIGHTS

Consider outfitting your personal gym in the cleaning supplies section of a grocery store. Many liquid detergents, bleaches, and fabric softeners are packaged in small plastic jugs with handles that fit rather conveniently into your hand. And the same product likely comes in varying sizes—50, 40, and 30 fluid ounces—which means you can have a nice collection of weights for incrementing and decrementing loads. When we work out with cleaning supplies, we call it "Clean and Jerk with Pride and Joy."

One client excitedly informed us that he was working out with a 50-ounce bottle. With 16 ounces to the pound, that's a little over three pounds! We hated to tell him that 50 fluid ounces doesn't mean that the bottle weighs 50 ounces.

Here's a little refresher course in math. Bear with us. You're going to need this information if you shop for your weights in the grocery store. In the United States, descriptions of exactly how much product is in a package are determined by universally accepted criteria set by the International Bureau of Standard Weights and Measures. The key words here are "Weights and Measures"—a clear indicator that stuff is measured at least two ways: *how much it weighs* and *how much volume it occupies*. The problem is that we use the word "ounce" to describe both. It can be a little confusing. One fluid ounce doesn't necessarily equal one ounce of weight. For example, one fluid ounce of oil, which is very dense, will weigh more than one fluid ounce of water.

A LITTLE MORE FOOD FOR THOUGHT WHEN SELECTING WEIGHTS AT THE GROCERY STORE

Cans of food make marvelous weights as long as they are small enough to hold in your hand. Their weights are printed right on the label, and many are standardized at one pound or 15 ounces (close enough). Cans are permanently sealed and can be used forever; they won't spoil or break open. An added benefit is that, if you're hungry after your workout, you can have a little snack.

Plastic bottles of detergent, cleaning fluid, water, milk, or juice are easily held in your hands and readily available. Additionally, you will find plastic jugs in all shapes and sizes—with handles. It doesn't matter which ones you select, but keep them full. Words of wisdom to the thirsty: if you're tempted and drink from your workout bottle (assuming that you're not training with detergent), all kinds of bad things will happen. First, you'll decrease the weight you're lifting. Your workout will be shot. Second, when you're working out both sides of your body simultaneously, and one bottle is suddenly lighter than the other,

How Does Your Weight Measure Up?

You will want to weigh each selection to make sure you've got what you need. Here's a little cheat sheet to help you get the right stuff.

Your Workout Equipment	Size	What It REALLY Weighs (in Pounds)
From the laundry section:		
Downy Fabric Softener	20 fluid ounces (600 ml)	1.49
	64 fluid ounces (1.89 liters)	4.42
Surf Detergent (liquid)	100 fluid ounces (3.12 qts)	7.33
Wisk Liquid Laundry Detergent	50 fluid ounces (1.4 liters)	3.85
	200 fluid ounces (5.91 liters)	14.83
From the cleaning supplies section:		
Dow Antibacterial Disinfectant	32 fluid ounces (946 ml)	2.20
Cascade Dishwasher Gel	85 ounces (2.4 kg)	5.75
Palmolive Dishwasher Gel	50 ounces (1.14 kg)	3.38
Sunlight Dishwasher Gel	5 lbs, 5 oz. (2.40 kg)	5.6
From the grocery, dairy, and beverage sections:		
Heinz Tomato Ketchup	*40 ounces (1134 grams)	2.67
Hershey's Chocolate Syrup	48 ounces (1.36 kg)	3.22
Hunt's BBQ Sauce	4 lbs, 13.5 oz. (2.20 kg)	5.09
Milk	1 Gallon	8.78
Water	*33.8 fluid ounces (1 liter)	2.38
	*50.6 fluid ounces (1.5 liters)	3.45
Wesson Canola Oil	64 fluid ounces (l.89 liters)	4.05
	*38 fluid ounces (1.12 liters)	2.38

* Bottle has no handle, but is small enough to lift safely in your hand.

your workout will become uneven. And finally, the drop in volume will cause a slosh. The slosh will cause the weight to lurch as you lift it, and you'll get thrown off balance. Get yourself a third bottle of water and designate it as drinking water. Or wait until your lifting is complete before you drink from your workout bottles. One more tip: NEVER lift with glass. ALWAYS lift with plastic. And ALWAYS tighten up the top before you start your workout.

If I Had a Hammer

You can lift virtually anything as long as you decide that it's safe and efficient—and doesn't mind being lifted (which precludes sneaking up on your sleeping Schnauzer). There is no end to the ingenuity we've seen. Following is a list of common items that we know work well:

Hammer

Wrench

Frying pan

Large flashlight

Tire iron

You'll have to tip the scales with whatever you select, to make sure that you're lifting just enough, but not too much. When you're experienced, you'll be able to "feel" when the weight is right.

Bags of dried beans or rice are perfect ankle and wrist weights. When tied on with cord, they conform comfortably to the contours of your body.

NOTES TO TRAINERS

If you're helping someone work out with Active-Isolated Strength training, you're going to be privileged to enjoy a very nice human connection. Here are some guidelines for you to follow, to keep the experience mutually beneficial:

- Show up on time, ready to work. If your partner has made the commitment to work out, you need to remember that it isn't easy to carve out the time and overcome all the excuses. Honor that commitment with one of your own.

- Talk for a moment before the workout, to gather information that might give you insight into your partner's well-being. Try to spot relevant things that might affect the upcoming workout.

- Tune in to your partner completely and without distraction.

- Keep eye contact and watch for small facial movement that signals discomfort or stress.

- Keep good notes regarding workouts and progression.

- Help your partner hold form for safety and maximum benefit from the lift.

- Keep accurate counts for your partner.

- Be alert for breath-holding or panting.

- Know when to touch your partner to correct or assist, and when to keep your hands off.

- Be respectful, and keep the workout on a professional level.

- Be encouraging, but avoid repeating clichéd "trainer talk" like, "Lookin' good!" After a while, it sounds to your partner as shallow and meaningless as it is.

- Review progress and plans every single day you work out.

- And finally, NEVER discuss your workouts or your partner with anyone. Ever.

THE NO-EXCUSES MANDATE

Active-Isolated Strength is a no-excuses workout, so let's learn to deal with time crunches and bad excuses. We once had a client who asked us to cut through the confusing hype of infomercials and tell him, conclusively, which piece of equipment he should order to strengthen and flatten his abs. Money was no object. He wanted results, preferably yesterday. Jim knew the answer before the client had the question out of his mouth and his VISA card out of his wallet. Jim answered honestly, "You don't need to buy equipment. You only need crunches." The client roared back, "Don't tell *me* about crunches! If I wasn't *always* in a crunch, I'd have time for this fitness stuff!" So what happens when the only "crunch" in your life is time, and you have trouble making room in your schedule for fitness? Frankly, it's a frustrating conundrum for everyone. We are the absolute masters of time management technologies and time-saving gadgetry. Yet, the more time we save, the less we seem to have. Indeed, we've all figured out how to be busier and busier.

There's little time for exercise. Ironically, making time for regular exercise is more important than ever, because we no longer have to expend much physical energy to get our daily tasks done. There once was a time when having mashed potatoes for supper meant digging, carrying, washing, peeling, slicing, wood chopping, fire building, water fetching, pot hauling, cow milking, pepper grinding, salt shaking, and frenzied mashing. Today, having mashed potatoes for dinner means driving to a market in an air-conditioned or heated car, parking ten feet from the front door, dashing in, buying frozen potatoes, zipping them home, popping them into the microwave oven, waiting one minute, and serving them in disposable containers that get tossed out before dessert. Unarguably, streamlined efficiency is great, but the human body is designed to *work* for its supper . . . and for everything else. And we just don't anymore. Unless we reintroduce physical exercise into our daily routines, our bodies respond to a lifetime of lethargy by turning to sludge on us. Unfortunately, to date, no one has yet figured out how to design instant fitness to go along with instant potatoes. The good news is that we can replace the hard work of our ancestors with fitness programs that are great fun and yield great results.

Part II

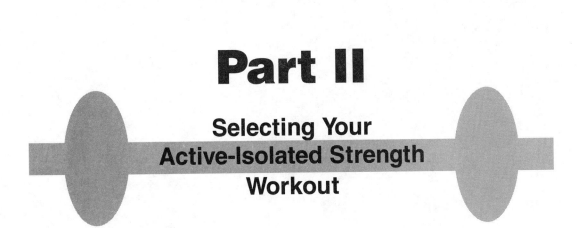

Selecting Your Active-Isolated Strength Workout

This is it! Time to roll up our sleeves and get to work.

It's important to understand that there is no magic. There are no quick fixes or easy answers in human performance. You have to get out there every day and *do* it. And you will, because you love it and it's your life. Somewhere along the way, you made a decision to be the best, and you have always known what it takes to get there and stay there. Active-Isolated Strength offers you a unique tool, but it's up to you to use it. We ask you to commit to the program for twenty-one days because we know that you'll form a habit in that amount of time. Anyone can do anything for three short weeks. At the end of that time, your athletic performance will be so improved and you'll feel so great that you won't want to quit.

Trust Us: Getting Started Is the Hardest Part

1. Make a decision to put Active-Isolated Strength training into your daily routine. Make that decision *once,* not again and again. For example, decide that you are going to get up twenty minutes earlier every morning so that you can get a workout. Decide that ONCE. Don't renegotiate it every morning. The alarm goes off, and you get up. No discussion, no whining.

2. Make a commitment. Make a deal with yourself to work out faithfully for twenty-one days. Being good at your sport has taught you to follow through. Now, you've made yourself a promise. No excuses. Follow through.

3. Do it. Show up on time, know the routine, get down and do it. Simple.

Get tough! The rewards of Active-Isolated Strength far outweigh the inconveniences of integrating a short new routine into your life. This book is a step-by-step guide that gives you techniques and tools developed over many years in sports clinics, venues, and training camps all over the world. Together, we'll help you reach your maximum performance potential.

Let's Get Started!

Zone 1

Upper Legs, Hips, and Trunk
(The Foundation)

1 Quadriceps—Knee Extensors

What You Strengthen:	The four muscles that form the strongest group in the body—the quadriceps ("quad" group) in the front of the thigh, from the top of the knee to the groin (vastus medialus, vastus intermedius, vastus lateralis, and rectus femoris)—plus sartorius and tensor fascia latae.
The Action:	Leg (knee) extension.
Equipment You Need:	Rolled towel or small pillow, ankle weight(s).

The Workout:

Put a weight on one ankle. Sit on a flat surface that allows your feet to be flat on the floor. Keep your back straight. Work one leg at a time. Tuck a rolled towel or a small pillow under the back of the knee of your exercising leg to take the pressure off your back and to elevate your foot so that it dangles slightly. Tighten your abdominal muscles to stabilize your trunk. Point your toes toward your nose. Contract your quadriceps to extend your leg straight out. Lock your knee. Hold for five seconds to contract the medial head of the vastus medialus—the insert of the small muscle at the top of the kneecap, on the inside of the thigh. (Strengthening this particular muscle attachment of the quadriceps group is important in stabilizing the knee, yet is overlooked if you fail to lock and hold for five seconds.) Return slowly to the starting position.

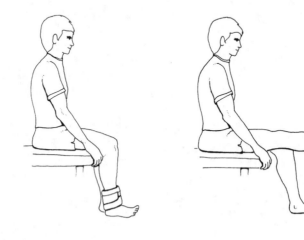

Managing Your Sets:

Lift 10 reps with your right leg. Then transfer the weight and lift 10 reps with your left leg. The combined twenty reps constitute one set. There is no need to rest if you alternate legs, unless you feel fatigued. The quads are two-joint muscles that extend the knee and flex the hip. Because each function needs to be isolated for a workout, you'll find one more quad lift in the workout program: Exercise 2, Quadriceps—Hip Flexors.

How long does it take when Jim and Phil work out?	
First Set:	2 minutes, 20 seconds
Second Set:	2 minutes, 20 seconds
Third Set:	2 minutes, 20 seconds
Total Time:	7 minutes

Taking It to the Gym:

Use any machine designed for leg extension or quadriceps strengthening. Strengthen *one leg at a time,* even if the machine is designed to work both legs simultaneously. Why? If one leg's quadriceps muscles are stronger than the other leg's, they'll compensate for the weaker muscles. Consequently, when both are worked simultaneously, the stronger leg will get stronger, and the weaker leg will never catch up. The difference may be subtle at first, and you may not even notice it, but the result could create significant imbalance and injury later. If you've been lifting with both legs and you correct your workout to engage only one leg at a time, be sure to decrease the weight you're lifting by 50 percent.

Some machines—particularly cams—lock your leg into a fixed position that doesn't allow natural tracking of the knee joint as you move. This can cause irritation. If you notice discomfort, try pulley machines or ankle weights.

2 Quadriceps—Hip Flexors

What You Strengthen:	The muscles in the front of the thigh, from the top of the knee to the groin (the quad group: vastus medialus, vastus intermedius, vastus lateralis, and rectus femoris) plus iliacus, sartorius, tensor fascia latae, gracilis, iliopsoas, and adductor magnus.
The Action:	Hip flexion.
Equipment You Need:	Ankle weight(s).

The Workout:

This exercise has three distinctive parts. Each part works the origins (upper attachments) of specific large and small muscles, on the front, inside, and outside of your thigh, respectively.

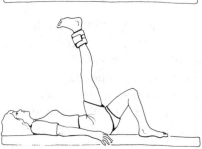

PART ONE (FRONT): Lie on your back on a flat surface. Strap a weight around the ankle of your exercising leg. Fully extend the leg. Lock your knee. Keep your foot relaxed and neutral (angled neither in nor out). Bend your nonexercising leg at the knee and place your foot flat on the surface to keep pressure off your back. From your hip and using your quadriceps, lift your leg straight up toward your head as far as you can. Aim the bottom of your foot toward the ceiling. Your goal should be to position your leg perpendicular to your body. Return slowly to the starting position.

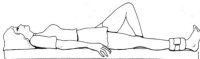

PART TWO (INSIDE): Without adjusting your basic position, turn out your exercising leg from your hip and point your toes to the outside. Keep your knee locked. From your hip and contracting your front and inner thigh muscles, lift your leg straight up toward your head as far as you can. Aim the bottom of your foot toward the ceiling. Return slowly to the starting position. This isolates the muscles on the *inside* of your upper thigh.

PART THREE (OUTSIDE): Again, without adjusting your basic position, turn in your exercising leg from your hip by pointing your toes to the inside. Keep your knee locked. From your hip and contracting your front and outer thigh muscles, lift your leg straight up toward your head as far as you can. Aim the bottom of your foot toward the ceiling. Return slowly to the starting position. This isolates the muscles on the *outside* of your upper thigh.

Managing Your Sets:

Because the positions of these lifts are very similar, it's efficient to combine them. Lift one rep front, one rep inside, one rep outside. Front, inside, outside. Front, inside, outside. Front. This is ten lifts on one leg in combination. Switch to the other side. There is no need to rest in between if you exercise alternate legs, unless you feel fatigued. One set of reps on the left leg and one set of reps on the right leg constitute one set.

How long does it take when Jim and Phil work out?	
First Set:	2 minutes, 20 seconds
Second Set:	2 minutes, 20 seconds
Third Set:	2 minutes, 20 seconds
Total Time:	7 minutes

Taking It to the Gym:

Use any machine designed for hip flexion. Strengthen *one* leg at a time, even if the machine is designed to work both legs simultaneously. Why? If one leg's quadriceps muscles are stronger than the other leg's, they'll compensate for the weaker muscles. Consequently, if you work both simultaneously, the stronger leg will get stronger, and the weaker leg will never catch up. The difference may be subtle at first, and you may not even notice it, but the result could create imbalance and injury later. If the machine locks both legs into position, totally relax one leg and allow the other to do all the work. If you've been lifting with both legs, and you correct your workout to engage only one leg at a time, be sure to decrease the weight you're lifting by 50 percent.

Be cautious when you use machines that encourage increasing weight by incrementing their loads ten pounds at a time with standard weight plates. Going from ten pounds to twenty pounds is an increase of 100 percent—far too much pressure and resistance for specific muscle attachments at that angle. Remember that you are lifting with smaller muscles when you lift your entire leg from your hip. Here, small amounts of weight make big differences.

3 *Hamstrings*

What You Strengthen:	The muscles in the rear of the thigh, from behind the knee to the buttocks (biceps femoris, semitendinosus, semimembranosus).
The Action:	Leg flexion.
Equipment You Need:	Ankle weight.

The Workout:

This exercise has three different positions within each set. Each isolates three primary muscles that make up the hamstring at the attachment above the knee. Work out one leg at a time.

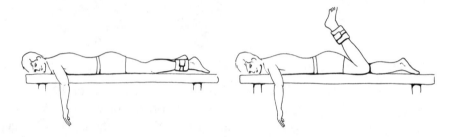

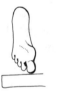

POSITION ONE (STRAIGHT): Lie on your stomach on a flat surface. Bring your foot toward your buttocks by contracting your hamstring muscles. Keep your hips flat and your foot straight. Return slowly to the starting position. This isolates the muscles in the middle of the rear thigh.

POSITION TWO (INSIDE): Without adjusting your position, turn your exercising foot out. Bring your foot toward your buttocks by contracting your hamstring muscles. Keep your hips flat and your foot turned out. Return slowly to the starting position. This isolates the muscles on the *inside* of the rear thigh.

POSITION THREE (OUTSIDE): Again, without adjusting your position, turn your exercising foot in. Bring your foot toward your buttocks by contracting your hamstring muscles. Keep your hips flat and your foot turned in. Return slowly to the starting position. This isolates the muscles on the *outside* of the rear thigh.

Managing Your Sets:

Because the positions of these lifts are very similar, it's efficient to combine them. Lift one rep straight, one rep inside, one rep outside. Straight, inside, outside. Straight, inside, outside. Straight. This is ten lifts on one leg in combination. Switch to the other side.

How long does it take when Jim and Phil work out?	
First Set:	2 minutes
Second Set:	2 minutes
Third Set:	2 minutes
Total Time:	6 minutes

Taking It to the Gym:

Be careful of machines that lock you into a fixed position, inhibit natural tracking of your muscles, and rob you of an effective workout. Also, the resistance provided by some machines is inconsistent as you run the range of motion on an exercise. Remember, strengthen *one* leg at a time, even if the machine is designed to work both legs simultaneously. If you've been lifting with both legs and you correct your workout to engage only one, be sure to decrease the weight you're lifting by 50 percent.

Some machines—particularly cams—lock your leg into a fixed position that doesn't allow natural tracking of the knee joint as you move. This can cause irritation. If you notice discomfort, try pulley machines or ankle weights.

4 Hip Extensors—Hamstrings

What You Strengthen:	The muscles in the rear of the thigh that attach to the "sit" bone (biceps femoris, semitendinosus and semimembranosus at the ischial tuberosity).
The Action:	Hip extension.
Equipment You Need:	Ankle weight.

The Workout:

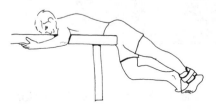

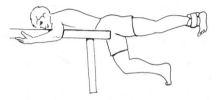

Lean forward over a workout table or bed with your pelvis at the edge, your stomach on the surface, and your feet on the floor. Put an ankle weight on your exercising leg. Bend your nonexercising leg to a 90-degree angle and let it relax. It should stabilize you, but not support your weight. Straighten your exercising leg and turn it in at the hip. With your foot turned toward the midline of your body, move your exercising leg toward the ceiling to the point where the buttocks muscles engage, but not beyond where it is parallel with your back and pelvis. (*Hyperextension* means going beyond normal range of motion. In some cases, it's acceptable, but with hamstring strengthening, it can strain your back.)

Managing Your Sets:

Lift one leg for ten reps and then lift the other leg for ten reps. This constitutes one set. It isn't necessary to rest between sets when you alternate legs, unless you're fatigued.

How long does it take when Jim and Phil work out?	
First Set:	2 minutes
Second Set:	2 minutes
Third Set:	2 minutes
Total Time:	6 minutes

Taking It to the Gym:

It's best to perform this exercise on a vertical (overhead) or a horizontal (standing) pulley machine. Your muscles can then track naturally, and you can increase your range of motion with each repetition. Remember to stabilize your body and keep your nonexercising leg relaxed so that you will not strain your back. If you have a choice, select the vertical machine.

5 Hip Abductors

What You Strengthen:	The muscles in the front of the thigh, from the top of the knee to the groin (tensor fascia latae, gluteus medius, vastus lateralis, and iliotibial band).
The Action:	Hip abduction.
Equipment You Need:	Rolled towel or small pillow, ankle weight(s).

The Workout:

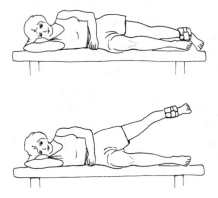

Put a weight on the ankle of your exercising leg. Lie on your side on a flat surface with both legs extended. Bend the knee of your bottom leg 90 degrees toward your chest, to stabilize your hips and take the pressure off your back. Keep the knee of your exercising leg straight. Lift your foot toward the ceiling, leading with your heel. This keeps your leg internally rotated. When you have gone as far as you can go (hopefully, to the point where your leg is nearly perpendicular to your body), hold for a moment and then return to the starting position.

Managing Your Sets:

Lift ten reps with one leg. Then roll over, transfer the weight to the other ankle, and lift the next ten reps with the opposite leg. This constitutes one set. There is no need to rest between sets if you alternate legs, unless you are feeling fatigued.

How long does it take when Jim and Phil work out?		
First Set:	1 minute,	40 seconds
Second Set:	1 minute,	40 seconds
Third Set:	1 minute,	40 seconds
Total Time:	5 minutes	

Taking It to the Gym:

Some machines—particularly cam machines with seats—lock your legs into a fixed position that doesn't allow natural tracking or proper isolation of the muscles. If you notice discomfort, try pulley machines or stay with your ankle weights.

6 Hip Adductors

What You Strengthen:	The muscles in the inside of the thigh, from the knee to the top of the groin area (adductor longus, adductor brevis, adductor magnus, and gracilis).
The Action:	Hip adduction.
Equipment You Need:	Ankle weight, a chair or coffee table.

The Workout:

Lie on your side on the floor. Put a weight on the ankle of your exercising (lower) leg. Extend both legs so your body forms a straight line. Keeping your knee straight, lift your top leg and rest your foot or ankle on some low, stable surface such as a chair or coffee table. Your leg should be at a 45-degree angle to the floor. Contract your abdominals to stay in alignment and to stop other muscle groups from compensating and assisting. Contract your inner thigh muscles and bring your bottom leg up to meet your top leg. Keep your knee locked. Slowly return to the starting position. Relax for an instant. Repeat.

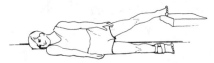 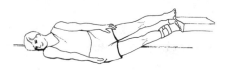

Managing Your Sets:

Lift ten reps with one leg. Then roll over, transfer the ankle weight, and lift the next ten reps with the opposite leg. Working both sides constitutes one set. There is no need to rest between sets if you alternate legs, unless you feel fatigued.

How long does it take when Jim and Phil work out?		
First Set:	1 minute,	30 seconds
Second Set:	1 minute,	30 seconds
Third Set:	1 minute,	30 seconds
Total Time:	4 minutes,	30 seconds

Taking It to the Gym:

It's best to perform this exercise on a vertical (overhead) or a horizontal (standing) pulley machine where your muscles can track naturally and where you can increase your range of motion with each repetition. Remember to stabilize your body and keep your nonexercising leg straight and relaxed so that you can maintain proper position. If you have a choice, select the vertical machine. Don't waste your time on any machine that requires you to sit. At that 90-degree angle (back up, legs out), your body will recruit adjacent muscles to assist the action, and you'll be unable to isolate the adductor from its hip attachment. So, although you "feel" muscles working, you're not getting full benefit.

7   *Gluteals*

What You Strengthen: Buttocks (gluteals—primarily gluteus maximus).
The Action: Hip extension with bent knee.
Equipment You Need: Ankle weights.

The Workout:

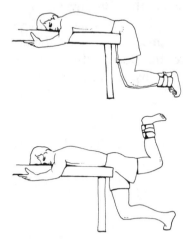

Bend over a bed or workout table with your pelvis on the edge and the ball of the foot of your nonexercising leg on the floor. Keep your nonexercising leg relaxed. Put an ankle weight on your exercising leg. Bend your exercising leg to 90 degrees and let it do all the work. (Resist the temptation to brace the foot of your nonexercising leg against the floor so you can push against it.) Move the exercising leg up toward the ceiling to the point where the buttocks muscles engage, but not beyond parallel with your back and pelvis.

Managing Your Sets:

Lift ten reps with one leg. Transfer the ankle weight, and lift the next ten reps with the opposite leg. Working both sides constitutes one set. There is no need to rest between sets if you alternate legs, unless you feel fatigued.

How long does it take when Jim and Phil work out?	
First Set:	50 seconds right
	50 seconds left
Second Set:	50 seconds right
	50 seconds left
Third Set:	50 seconds right
	50 seconds left
Total Time:	5 minutes

Taking It to the Gym:

Machines at the gym work well here, where a locked position helps isolate and track muscles properly. Be sure to use machines that allow you to work out one leg at a time and put no strain on your back.

8 Hip External Rotators

What You Strengthen:	Deep muscles in the buttocks that externally rotate the hips (gluteus maximus, obturator internus and externus, inferior and superior gemellus, and piriformis).
The Action:	Seated—lower leg internal rotation with external or lateral rotation of the femur.
Equipment You Need:	Ankle weight, rope, and a rolled towel or small pillow.

The Workout:

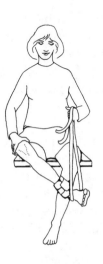

Sit on a bed or table with your lower legs dangling over the edge. Strap a weight on the ankle of your exercising leg. Tuck a rolled towel or a small pillow under your knee. Loop your rope around the arch of the foot of the exercising leg, with the loose ends to the inside. Reach down and grasp the rope with the hand on the opposite side of your body, and gently lift up to remove slack. Place your other hand (on the same side as your exercising leg) on the top of your thigh just above the knee and grasp the muscle with your thumb, to stabilize your leg and to assist in the rotation. Now, rotate the lower part of your exercising leg toward the midline of your body. Go as far as you can. At the point when you are no longer able to continue the upward pendulumlike swing of your lower leg, gently assist by pulling upward on the rope to extend your range of motion. Added benefit: you'll get a good Active-Isolated Stretch. Relax the tension on the rope and slowly return to the starting position. Repeat.

Managing Your Sets:

Lift one leg for ten reps and then lift the other leg for ten reps. This constitutes one set. It isn't necessary to rest between sets when you alternate legs, unless you're fatigued.

How long does it take when Jim and Phil work out?	
First Set:	2 minutes
Second Set:	2 minutes
Third Set:	2 minutes
Total Time:	6 minutes

Taking It to the Gym:

Go into the free weight room and strap on an ankle weight.

9 *Hip Internal Rotators*

What You Strengthen:	Deep muscles in the top of the buttocks that internally rotate the hips (gluteus minimus and medius), the muscles that span the hip sockets to the top of the pelvis (tensor fascia latae), and the muscles that reach from the bottom front of the pelvis to the inside of the thighs, halfway down the femur (adductors).
The Action:	Seated—lower leg external rotation of the lower leg with internal rotation of the femur.
Equipment You Need:	Ankle weight, rope, and a rolled towel or small pillow.

The Workout:

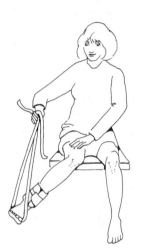

Sit on a bed or table with your lower legs dangling over the edge. Tuck a rolled towel or a small pillow under your knee. Loop your rope around the arch of the foot of your exercising leg, with the loose ends to the outside. Reach down and grasp the rope with the hand on the same side of your body, and gently lift up to remove slack. Place your other hand on the top of your thigh just above the knee and grasp the muscle with your thumb, to stabilize your leg, keep it from lifting, and assist in the rotation. Now, rotate the lower part of your exercising leg away from the midline of your body. Go as far as you can. At the point when you are no longer able to continue the upward pendulumlike swing of your lower leg, gently assist by pulling up on the rope to extend your range of motion. Added benefit: you'll get a good Active-Isolated Stretch. Relax the tension on the rope and slowly return to the starting position.

Managing Your Sets:

Lift one leg for ten reps, then lift the other leg for ten reps. This constitutes one set. There is no need to rest between sets, unless you feel fatigued.

How long does it take when Jim and Phil work out?	
First Set:	2 minutes
Second Set:	2 minutes
Third Set:	2 minutes
Total Time:	6 minutes

Taking It to the Gym:

Go into the free weight room and strap on an ankle weight.

10 Sacrospinalis

What You Strengthen:	Lower back (sacrospinalis and erector spinae).
The Action:	Double-leg hip extension.
Equipment You Need:	Ankle weight.

The Workout:

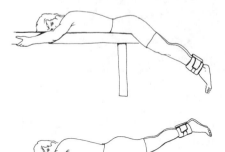

Put your feet together and fasten one ankle weight around both ankles. Bend over a bed or table with your pelvis on the edge and your feet on the floor. Grip the edge of the bed or table to stabilize your body, and lift your legs (knees straight and locked!) toward the ceiling, leading with your heels. Lift as far as you can go. Hold for a moment, and then slowly lower your legs until your toes touch the floor.

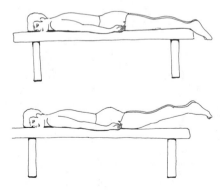

Note: If your back is weak, lie flat on your abdomen on a surface that supports your body down to your ankles. Place your arms at your sides. Relax everything above your waist. Straighten your legs and point your toes. Lock your knees. Lift your legs gently off the surface until you feel the muscles in your buttocks (glutes) contract. Lift as far as you can without discomfort. Your back is not involved. Hold for a moment and then slowly lower your legs back to the starting position.

Managing Your Sets:

Lift both legs together ten times. This constitutes one set.

How long does it take when Jim and Phil work out?	
First Set:	30 seconds
Rest:	*30 seconds*
Second Set:	30 seconds
Rest:	*30 seconds*
Third Set:	30 seconds
Total Time:	2 minutes, 30 seconds

Taking It to the Gym:

This time, it's better to use your own body and sensibilities than to search for equipment.

11 Upper Abdominals

What You Strengthen:	Muscles in the upper abdomen (rectus abdominus, transversus abdominis, linea alba).
The Action:	Trunk flexion with bent knees.
Equipment You Need:	Heavy furniture to hold your feet down. When you are advanced, you can hold an ankle weight in your hands, against your chest, to add more resistance.

The Workout:

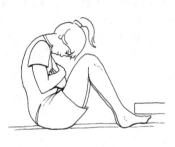

Lie flat on your back. Bend your knees and lock your feet under something heavy—like a couch—that will help you keep them firmly down. Fold your hands across your chest, and tuck your chin in. This tucking will lift your head off the surface and begin the rolling action you need to isolate and fire the abdominal muscles at the sternum, and to block your body's attempt to recruit other muscles to assist. Roll up slowly until you are upright and your chest is at your knees. Hold for a moment and then roll slowly back down, placing one vertebra at a time on the floor surface until your head is back down. Relax for a moment and then resume an upward roll. If you have too little "natural padding" on your tailbone, be certain to spread a towel under your fanny.

Note: If your back is too weak to do this exercise as we have described it, you can modify the moves. If you are able, tuck your chin until your shoulders leave the surface and you feel your abdominals contract. Keep your back flat on the surface. Hold for a moment. Then relax, slowly lowering your head.

Managing Your Sets:

Rest thirty seconds between sets.

How long does it take when Jim and Phil work out?	
First Set:	1 minute	
Rest:		*30 seconds*
Second Set:	1 minute	
Rest:		*30 seconds*
Third Set:	1 minute	
Total Time:	4 minutes, 30 seconds	

Taking It to the Gym:

Experts agree that abdominal rollers or crunching machines are not as effective as good old-fashioned "sit-ups" on the floor. Machines can leave you open to a couple of potential risks: (1) they allow your body to recruit assistance from muscles other than your abdominals, making your workout less effective, and (2) they can strain your back.

12 Oblique Abdominals

What You Strengthen:	Muscles on the sides of the abdomen (rectus abdominis, internal and external obliques, transversus abdominis).
The Action:	Bent-knee trunk flexion with rotation.
Equipment You Need:	Heavy furniture to hold your feet down. When you are advanced, you can hold an ankle weight in your hands, against your chest, to add more resistance.

The Workout:

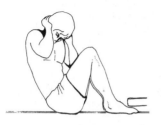

Lie flat on your back. Bend your knees and lock your feet under something heavy—like a couch—that will help you keep them firmly down. Tuck your chin in. Interlace your hands behind your head. Twist your torso to one side. Lead with your elbow and roll up slowly until you're upright or can go no further. Hold for a moment and then, still in rotation, roll slowly back down, setting one vertebra at a time on the surface until your head is back down. Relax for a moment and then resume a twist and an upward roll. If you have too little "natural padding" on your tailbone, spread a towel under your buttocks.

Note: If your back is weak or injured, you can modify this exercise. If you are able, tuck your chin and twist until your shoulders leave the surface and you feel your obliques contract. Keep your back flat on the surface. Hold for a moment. You'll feel your obliques working. Then, slowly lower your head and untwist.

Managing Your Sets:

Alternate sides as you work out: left, right, left, right, and so on. Rest thirty seconds between sets.

How long does it take when Jim and Phil work out?		
First Set:	1 minute,	30 seconds
Rest:		*30 seconds*
Second Set:	1 minute,	30 seconds
Rest:		*30 seconds*
Third Set:	1 minute,	30 seconds
Total Time:	5 minutes,	30 seconds

Taking It to the Gym:

Experts agree that abdominal rollers or crunching machines are not as effective as good old-fashioned "sit-ups" on the floor. Machines can leave you open to a couple of potential risks: (1) they allow your body to recruit assistance from muscles other than your abdominals, diluting the effectiveness of your workout, and (2) they can strain your back.

13 Lower Abdominals

What You Strengthen:	Muscles in the lower abdomen (lower rectus abdominis, pyramidalis, linea alba, and stabilizers such as obturator internus).
The Action:	Reverse curl-up.
Equipment You Need:	When you're advanced, you can use an ankle weight strapped around both ankles.

The Workout:

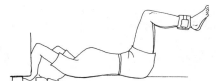

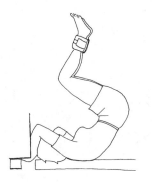

Lie flat on your back. Bend your knees. Put your feet flat and press your ankles together. This will focus your center of gravity, give you added stability, and enhance your ability to isolate muscles. Reach over your head and lock your hands under something heavy—like a couch—that will support your weight. Roll your knees up until your upper legs are perpendicular to the surface and your lower legs are parallel to the surface. When you are into this "launch" position, project your knees straight up toward the ceiling. Your buttocks will follow and you'll feel your lower abdominals engage. When you're up as far as you can go and you're supported by your shoulders, then allow your body to roll forward slightly. Hold for a moment and then return slowly to the starting position. Remember, keep your knees bent, and resist the temptation to arch your back. If you have too little "natural padding" on your tailbone, spread a towel under your fanny.

If you are unable to lift your torso to the ceiling from the launch position, work up to it slowly. Merely contract your lower abdominals to a point where you can lift your buttocks from the surface slightly. Be patient. You'll get stronger.

Note: If your back is weak or injured, you can modify this exercise. Lie flat on your back. Bend your knees and place your feet flat. Keep your back on the surface, contract your lower abdominals, tilt your pelvis slightly, and lift your buttocks two to three inches. Hold for a moment. Slowly return to starting position. Relax. (If you like, you can place an ankle weight on your abdomen, right below your belly button, for a little more resistance.)

Managing Your Sets:

Lift your legs ten times per set. Rest thirty seconds between sets.

How long does it take when Jim and Phil work out?	
First Set:	1 minute
Rest:	*30 seconds*
Second Set:	1 minute
Rest:	*30 seconds*
Third Set:	1 minute
Total Time:	4 minutes

Taking It to the Gym:

Use a bench with a belt, for leverage.

14 Trunk Extensors and Rotators

What You Strengthen:	Muscles in the sides of your back (external obliques).
The Action:	Full spinal extension and flexion in rotation.
Equipment You Need:	Technically, a person is not "equipment." You need a helper with this workout.

The Workout:

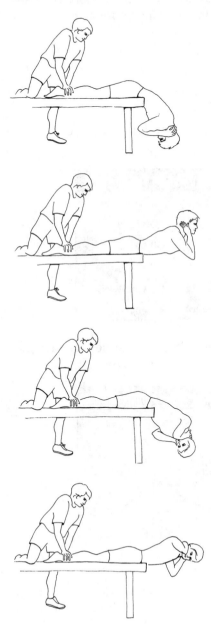

You can't do this one alone! Lie flat on your stomach, on a bed or a table, and hang over the edge from your waist up. (In other words, your legs and pelvis will be on the surface and your upper body will be dangling.) Your helper must hold your lower legs or ankles to keep you from sliding onto the floor and to give you leverage so you can lift your own weight without flipping off. Place your hands on your cheeks and tuck your elbows in tight. (Tucking your elbows in immobilizes the traps and rhomboids—two muscle groups that rush to assist a lazy and ever-weakening mid and lower back.) Relax and tuck your head down. Lift straight up. This works out your extensors. Slowly return to starting position. Rotate your upper torso to one side as far as you can and hold that position. Now, lift your upper body up from your waist until you're cantilevered straight out. Hold your position in rotation. This works out your rotators. Slowly lower yourself back to the starting position. Twist to the other side and repeat.

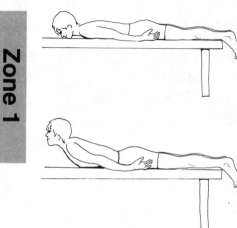

Note: If your back is weak, you can modify this exercise. Lie flat on your stomach with your arms at your sides. Relax everything below your waist. Lift your head and chest off the surface and roll your shoulders back as far as you're able without discomfort. Your back will be arched. Hold for a moment and then slowly lower yourself back to the starting position.

Managing Your Sets:

For extensors, lift upper body straight up ten times. This constitutes one set.

How long does it take when Jim and Phil work out?	
First Set:	30 seconds
Rest:	*30 seconds*
Second Set:	30 seconds
Rest:	*30 seconds*
Third Set:	30 seconds
Total Time:	2 minutes, 30 seconds

For rotators, lift your upper body ten times on each side (alternating left and right). This constitutes one set.

How long does it take when Jim and Phil work out?	
First Set:	1 minute
Rest:	*30 seconds*
Second Set:	1 minute
Rest:	*30 seconds*
Third Set:	1 minute
Total Time:	4 minutes

Taking It to the Gym:

Use a Roman chair or a bench designed to hold your legs in a fixed position while you cantilever your body up and out.

15 Trunk Lateral Flexors

What You Strengthen:	Sides of back (quadratus lumborum, deep posterior rotators and external obliques).
The Action:	Lateral trunk flexion.
Equipment You Need:	Technically, a person is not "equipment." You need a helper with this workout.

The Workout:

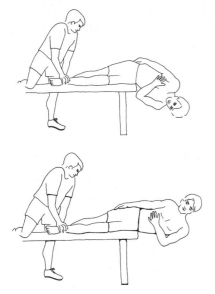

"Good-bye, love handles!" Lie on your side on a bed or a table. While a partner holds your lower calves and ankles, scoot over the edge until you are cantilevered off the surface from your waist up. Keep your top arm and hand straight and on your side. Fold your bottom arm and hand over your chest. Bend down with your head toward the floor. Remember to keep your body relaxed and in alignment. Go down as far as possible from the starting position. You'll feel a stretch along your side. Slowly lift your upper torso back up until your body is back in a straight line. Repeat.

Managing Your Sets:

Ten reps constitutes one set. Take a 30-second rest between sets.

How long does it take when Jim and Phil work out?	
First Set:	1 minute
Rest:	*30 seconds*
Second Set:	1 minute
Rest:	*30 seconds*
Third Set:	1 minute
Total Time:	4 minutes

Taking It to the Gym:

Use a Roman chair. If you must cross your legs in order to get into position on the chair, put your top leg behind you to keep you from rolling.

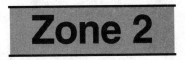

Zone 2

Shoulders

16 Deltoids

What You Strengthen:	Front of shoulders (anterior deltoid, clavicular head of pectoralis major and coracobrachialis), upper back and middle shoulders (supraspinatus and deltoid), and back of shoulders and upper arms (posterior deltoid, latissimus dorsi, and teres major).
The Action:	In sequence: forward elevation (flexion), sideways elevation (abduction), and backward elevation (extension) of the shoulder group.
Equipment You Need:	One or two handheld weights (dumbbells).

The Workout:

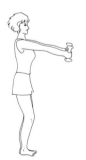

This workout is done in three parts.

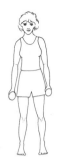

PART ONE (WORKS THE FRONT OF THE SHOULDERS): You can sit or stand. If you're standing, slightly bend your knees and contract your abdominals to protect your back from hyperextension. Grasp your weights. You can lift with both shoulders at the same time, but if you do, make certain that the weights are the same in both hands. With your arms straight at your sides, slowly bring the weight straight up in front of you to shoulder level. Hold for a moment and then return to the starting position.

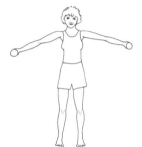

PART TWO (WORKS THE UPPER BACK AND MIDDLE SHOULDER): Stay in position. With your arms hanging straight down, the palms of your hands facing toward the midline of your body, and your elbows locked, slowly bring the weights out to the sides and up to shoulder level. Resist the urge to hike your shoulders up. Hold for a moment and then return to the starting position.

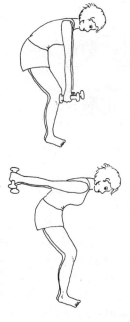

PART THREE (WORKS THE BACK OF THE SHOULDERS AND UPPER ARMS): Stay in position. Bend forward at the waist until your chest is at about a 45-degree angle to the floor. With your arms hanging straight down, the palms of your hands facing toward the midline of your body, and your elbows locked, slowly bring the weight backward and up as far as possible toward shoulder level (and higher if you can). Hold for a moment and then return to the starting position.

Managing Your Sets:

As you lift, alternate the lifts: forward elevation, sideways elevation, backward elevation; forward, sideways, backward; and so on. When you have completed ten of each of the three lifts in sequence, this constitutes one set. There is no need to rest between sets, unless you feel fatigued.

How long does it take when Jim and Phil work out?		
First Set:	1 minute,	20 seconds
Second Set:	1 minute,	20 seconds
Third Set:	1 minute,	20 seconds
Total Time:	4 minutes	

Taking It to the Gym:

You can use a pulley machine with a cable and a handle. It might be necessary to bend forward at the waist, and swing your arm up and back. Put one foot in front of the other to provide yourself with more stability and less pressure on your back. Put the hand of your nonexercising arm on your exercising thigh to brace your body into position.

17 *Pectoralis Major*

What You Strengthen:	Chest front (pectoralis major and minor, and anterior deltoid).
The Action:	Straight arm (horizontal) adduction.
Equipment You Need:	Two handheld weights (dumbbells or ankle weights held in your hands).

The Workout:

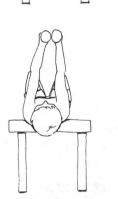

Lie down on your back with your knees bent and your feet flat. Extend your arms out to your sides with your elbows locked, your palms up, and a weight in each hand. It's best to lift from both sides at the same time. And remember, the weights should be equal. Bring your hands straight up toward the ceiling, and have the weights meet above your face. Return slowly to the starting position.

Managing Your Sets:

Ten reps constitute one set. Plan to rest 30 seconds between each set. This lift works really well in combination with Exercise 18, Triceps—Supine. As long as you're already on your back with weights in your hands, plan to transition from this lift right into the next one.

How long does it take when Jim and Phil work out?	
First Set:	40 seconds
Rest:	*30 seconds*
Second Set:	40 seconds
Rest:	*30 seconds*
Third Set:	40 seconds
Total Time:	3 minutes

Zone 2

Taking It to the Gym:

You can use a double pulley machine with a cable and a handle. Choose machines that promote the full range of motion and approximate the natural tracking of muscles (such as swinging a tennis racket). Avoid machines that abbreviate the action or put your arms into shortened angles. A workout on one of them may seem like a good one, but you'll soon discover that not all muscles are created equal. You might be able to develop the bellies of the large muscles, but unhappily discover that the attachments of the smaller muscles are weak and blow out when they're stressed.

Zone 2

18 *Triceps—Supine*

What You Strengthen:	Muscles in the back of the upper arm (triceps brachii—medial head).
The Action:	Elbow extension.
Equipment You Need:	Two handheld weights (dumbbells or ankle weights held in your hands).

The Workout:

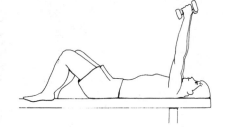

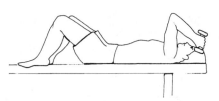

Lie down on your back with your knees bent and your feet flat. Start by holding the weights up perpendicular to the floor, with your palms facing each other, your elbows locked and straight over your shoulders. Bring the weights down by keeping your upper arm straight up and flexing your elbows until the weights are near the surface on either side of your head. Hold for a moment. Return slowly to the starting position.

Caution: Stay alert during this exercise! Working out with weight suspended over your face could result in more "iron" in your diet than you planned. You know what we mean.

Managing Your Sets:

Ten reps constitute one set. Plan to rest 30 seconds between each set. This lift works really well in combination with Exercise 17, Pectoralis Major. As long as you're already on your back with weights in your hands, plan to transition from that lift right into this one.

How long does it take when Jim and Phil work out?	
First Set:	20 seconds
Rest:	*30 seconds*
Second Set:	20 seconds
Rest:	*30 seconds*
Third Set:	20 seconds
Total Time: 2 minutes	

Taking It to the Gym:

You'll do best if you can use a seated cam machine that stabilizes your position and tracking with padding. If a cam is not available, you can use a pulley machine with a cable and a bar in front of you, but you need to be aware that, when you work with both arms simultaneously on a bar, the stronger arm will do most of the work and the weaker arm will allow it. You'll never know the difference. But, as a consequence, your weaker arm will stay weaker and will never balance. Also, if you are not in perfect alignment, other muscles will tighten up—particularly in your back—to help you get that bar down. With pulley machines, lying down is better than sitting, and sitting is better than standing.

Zone 2

19 Shoulder External Rotators

What You Strengthen:	Deep shoulder or rotator cuff (infraspinatus, teres minor, and supraspinatus).
The Action:	Shoulder external rotation.
Equipment You Need:	One or two handheld weights (dumbbells), or ankle weights held in your hands.

The Workout:

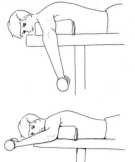

Lie down on your abdomen on a bed or a table with your exercising arm dangling off the edge and a weight in your hand. Turn your head to one side and relax your neck. Place a rolled-up towel under the front of your shoulder. Bring your elbow to a 90-degree angle, with your knuckles facing forward. (You can work out both sides at the same time. Just make sure the weights are equal.) Bring your bent arm straight up until your knuckles are level with your head. Hold for a moment. Return slowly to the starting position.

Caution: Keep your elbow at 90 degrees to keep the weight away from your face as you bring it up. Nothing ruins a good workout like a broken nose.

Managing Your Sets:

Ten reps of each arm constitutes one set. Plan to rest 30 seconds between each set. This lift works really well in combination with Exercise 20, Shoulder Internal Rotators, and Exercise 21, Triceps—Prone Position. As long as you're already on your abdomen with weights in your hands, plan to transition from this lift right into the next one.

How long does it take when Jim and Phil work out?	
First Set:	**20 seconds**
Rest:	*30 seconds*
Second Set:	**20 seconds**
Rest:	*30 seconds*
Third Set:	**20 seconds**
Total Time:	**2 minutes***
***Both sides worked simultaneously.**	

Taking It to the Gym:

This is a light-weight exercise. Minor muscles are always used, but seldom strengthened. We think free weights are best.

20 *Shoulder Internal Rotators*

What You Strengthen:	Deep shoulder or rotator cuff, and side of chest (subscapularis, teres major, and pectoralis major).
The Action:	Shoulder internal rotation.
Equipment You Need:	One or two handheld weights (dumbbells), or ankle weights held in your hands.

The Workout:

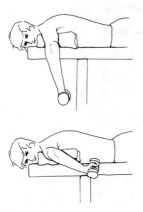

Lie down on your abdomen on a bed or a table with your exercising arm dangling off the edge and a weight in your hand. Turn your head to one side and relax your neck. Place a rolled-up towel under the front of your shoulder to take the strain off the clavicular head of your pectoralis muscles. Bring your elbow to a 90-degree angle, with your knuckles facing forward. (You can work out both sides at the same time if you're lying on a surface that's narrow enough—a bench, for example. Just make sure the weights are equal.) Lock your wrist and bring your hand straight back, leading with your palm as far as you can go. (Resist the generous offer of your back muscles to help your shoulder do its work. You'll know the offer has been made when your shoulder blade—scapula—cocks up and your elbow moves skyward.) Hold for a moment. Return slowly to the starting position.

Zone 2

Managing Your Sets:

Ten reps of each arm constitutes one set. Plan to rest 30 seconds between each set. This lift works really well in combination with Exercise 19, Shoulder External Rotators, and Exercise 21, Triceps—Prone Position. As long as you're already on your abdomen with weights in your hands, plan to transition from this lift right into the next one.

How long does it take when Jim and Phil work out?	
First Set:	20 seconds
Rest:	*30 seconds*
Second Set:	20 seconds
Rest:	*30 seconds*
Third Set:	20 seconds
Total Time: 2 minutes*	
*Both sides worked simultaneously.	

Taking It to the Gym:

This exercise is done with light weights. Minor muscles are always used, but seldom strengthened. We think free weights are best.

21 Triceps—Prone

What You Strengthen:	Muscles in the back of the upper arm (triceps brachii—long and lateral heads).
The Action:	Elbow extension.
Equipment You Need:	One or two handheld weights (dumbbells), or ankle weights held in your hands.

The Workout:

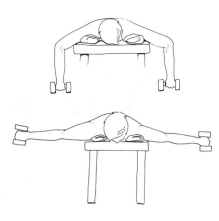

Lie down on your abdomen on a bed or a table. Have the upper part of your exercising arm(s) straight out from your body, dangle your forearm(s) off the edge, and hold the weight(s) in your hand(s). Turn your head to one side to take stress off your back and make breathing easier. Place a rolled-up towel under the front of your shoulder to take the strain off the clavicular head of your pectoralis muscles. (You can work out both sides at the same time if you're lying on a surface that's narrow enough—a bench, for example. Just make sure the weights are equal.) Your elbow should be at 90 degrees, with your knuckles facing forward. Bring your hand straight out and up until your elbow is locked. Hold for a moment. Return slowly to the starting position.

Managing Your Sets:

Ten reps of each arm constitutes one set. Plan to rest 30 seconds between each set. This lift works really well in combination with Exercise 19, Shoulder External Rotators, and Exercise 20, Shoulder Internal Rotators. As long as you're already on your abdomen with weights in your hands, plan to transition from those lifts right into this one.

How long does it take when Jim and Phil work out?	
First Set:	20 seconds
Rest:	*30 seconds*
Second Set:	20 seconds
Rest:	*30 seconds*
Third Set:	20 seconds
Total Time: 2 minutes*	
Both sides worked simultaneously.	

Zone 2

69

Taking It to the Gym:

You'll do best if you can use a cam machine that stabilizes your position and tracking with padding. If a cam is not available, you can use a pulley machine with a cable and a handle. No matter which you choose, just be sure the starting position of your arm is straight out from your body and your elbow is bent to a 90-degree angle, with your forearm down.

22 *Trapezius*

What You Strengthen:	Outer group of muscles that steadies and controls the upper back and the connection of the shoulder (trapezius, posterior deltoid, teres major and minor, supraspinatus, infraspinatus, and rhomboids).
The Action:	Shoulder abduction.
Equipment You Need:	Two handheld weights (dumbbells).

Zone 2

The Workout:

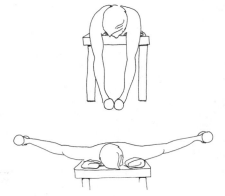

Lie down on your stomach on a bed or a table. Pull your body forward until you are suspended out as far as your armpits. You will be working both arms simultaneously. Dangle your arms straight down from your shoulders. Keep your head and neck aligned with your torso. Take one weight in each hand. (Remember, they must be equal.) Start with the weights right below your face. Hold your arms straight and your elbows locked. Leading with your knuckles, bring the weights out to your sides and up as far as you can go. Hold for a moment. Return slowly to the starting position.

Managing Your Sets:

Ten reps constitute one set. Plan to rest 30 seconds between each set. This lift works really well in combination with Exercise 23, Rhomboids. As long as you're already on your abdomen with weights in your hands, plan to transition from this lift right into that one.

How long does it take when Jim and Phil work out?	
First Set:	40 seconds
Rest:	*30 seconds*
Second Set:	40 seconds
Rest:	*30 seconds*
Third Set:	40 seconds
Total Time:	3 minutes

Taking It to the Gym:

You can stand, and use a cable and pulley system. Remember to bend forward 90 degrees at the waist, contract your abdominals to stabilize your body, and keep your back straight. You'll work one arm at a time. Place the hand of your nonexercising arm on the thigh of your exercising side to help your balance.

We think the seated machines can help you do the job, but they can put pressure on your back. Lying down to do the work is better than standing. And standing is better than sitting.

23   *Rhomboids*

What You Strengthen:	The inner group of muscles that steadies and controls the upper back, and the connection of the shoulder (rhomboids major and minor, supraspinatus, infraspinatus, levator scapulae, and pectoralis minor).
The Action:	Bent elbow, horizontal shoulder abduction.
Equipment You Need:	Two handheld weights (dumbbells).

The Workout:

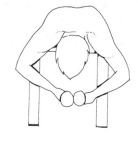

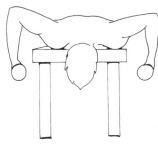

Lie down on your stomach on a bed or a table. Pull your body forward until you are suspended out as far as your armpits. You will be working both arms simultaneously. Dangle your arms down over the edge. Relax your neck so that your head drops down. Take one weight in each hand. (Remember, they must be equal.) Your palms should face up and your thumbs should point forward. Lock your elbows at 90-degree angles and touch the weights together in line with your nose. This is the starting position. Bring your locked elbows up toward the ceiling as far as you can go, separating the weights. Hold for a moment. Return slowly to the starting position.

Managing Your Sets:

Ten reps constitute one set. Plan to rest 30 seconds between each set. This lift works really well in combination with Exercise 22, Trapezius. As long as you're already on your abdomen with weights in your hands, plan to transition from that lift right into this one.

How long does it take when Jim and Phil work out?	
First Set:	40 seconds
Rest:	*30 seconds*
Second Set:	40 seconds
Rest:	*30 seconds*
Third Set:	40 seconds
Total Time: 3 minutes	

Zone 2

Taking It to the Gym:

You can stand, and use a cable and pulley system. Remember to bend forward 90 degrees at the waist, contract your abdominals to stabilize your body, relax your neck and drop your head, lock your elbows into 90-degree angles, and keep your back straight. You'll work one arm at a time. Place the hand of your nonexercising arm on the thigh of your exercising side to help your balance.

We think the seated machines can help you do the job, but they can put pressure on your back. Even though you're upright, keep your neck relaxed and your head down, to isolate the rhomboids and keep other muscles (like your trapezius) from engaging to help do the work. Lying down is better than standing. And standing is better than sitting.

24 Biceps

What You Strengthen:	Front of the upper arm (biceps brachii, brachialis, brachioradialis, extensor carpi radialis longus, and pronator teres).
The Action:	Elbow flexion.
Equipment You Need:	One or two handheld weights (dumbbells or ankle weights).

The Workout:

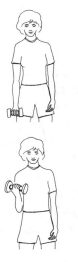

It really makes no difference whether you sit or stand, but we prefer standing. It's physiologically more efficient. As you progress to greater and greater weight, however, you may prefer sitting in order to help avoid putting pressure on your back. You can work both arms at the same time, but use individual weights rather than a barbell. Remember that the weights must be equal. Hold the weight in your hand with the palm up. Tuck your elbow tightly into your body between your hip bone and waist, so that you are stabilized and locked into proper position. Start with the weight down at your side. Keep your elbow straight and your wrist locked. Your palm should face your bicep. Contract your biceps and slowly bend your elbow to bring the weight straight up in front of you to your shoulder, keeping your elbow and upper arm tightly against your body.

Managing Your Sets:

Ten reps constitute one set. Plan to rest 30 seconds between each set if you lift with both arms simultaneously.

How long does it take when Jim and Phil work out?	
First Set:	30 seconds
Rest:	*30 seconds*
Second Set:	30 seconds
Rest:	*30 seconds*
Third Set:	30 seconds
Total Time:	2 minutes, 30 seconds

Taking It to the Gym:

Your first choice is a cable and pulley with a handle. Work one side at a time. You may stand, sit, or kneel.

Your second choice is a seated machine. However, you should be aware that the machine can do too much work for you. It may restrict your movements too much and impede your muscles' natural tracking.

Zone 2

25 *Shoulder (The Roll)*

What You Strengthen:	The inner group of muscles that steadies and controls the upper back, and the connection of the shoulder (rhomboids major and minor; trapezius; supraspinatus; infraspinatus; levator scapulae; serratus anterior; and subclavius).
The Action:	Rotating shoulders.
Equipment You Need:	Two handheld weights (dumbbells or ankle weights).

The Workout:

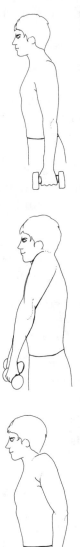

You need to work both shoulders at the same time. Stand with your back straight, feet slightly apart, knees slightly bent, and abdominals contracted for stability. Take a weight in each hand, with your palms facing in and your thumbs pointing forward. Relax your arms down at your sides. Straighten your elbows. Keep your spine straight and your head in line with your spine. In a continuous, slow, and controlled motion, roll your shoulders forward, up, over, back, under, and down. The sequence of action will be lateral abduction (roll forward), elevation (lift), medial adduction (roll backward), and inferior depression (letting your shoulders down). We'll tell you a little secret: the real power in this workout is in the backward roll, when you adduct the shoulder blades (scapula).

Note: This may very well be the world's greatest stress buster. When we hear "Oooo . . . ahhh . . . mmmm" from behind the closed door in our clinic, we can be certain that one of two great pleasures in life is going on . . . and it's probably the Shoulder Roll. This workout strengthens while it relaxes a real trouble spot for most people: the middle of the upper back. That unmistakable feeling that there's a rusty railroad spike embedded between your shoulder blades is a double whammy delivered by the back and shoulders. Here's how. The upper fibers of the back are generally oversolicited when people work, and the shoulder, ironically, is one of the most mobile and yet least stable of all the joints in the body. The combination can be stressful. Almost everyone complains of "carrying tension" between the shoulder blades, which leads to a tight back, headaches, and a stiff neck. This sensation isn't actually "carrying tension"; it's pain from weak muscles that have shorted out, gone into contraction, and locked up.

Managing Your Sets:

Ten reps constitute one set. Plan to rest 30 seconds between each set.

How long does it take when Jim and Phil work out?	
First Set:	40 seconds
Rest:	*30 seconds*
Second Set:	40 seconds
Rest:	*30 seconds*
Third Set:	40 seconds
Total Time:	3 minutes

Taking It to the Gym:

It's a free weight workout, but don't be tempted to use a single barbell instead of two dumbbells. If you've got a barbell in your hands, when you try to roll your shoulders back, the bar will smack up against your body and block the roll. You'll never get the full range of motion you need to get your shoulders back.

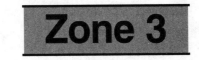

Zone 3

Neck

26 Neck Extensors, Flexors, and Rotators

What You Strengthen:	*Back* of the neck (erector spinae, splenius capitis, multifidus, and sternocleidomastoid), *sides* of the neck (sternocleidomastoid, splenius capitis, anterior scalene, levator scapulae, and trapezius), *muscles that help turn the head* (obliques capitis superior and inferior, rectus capitis posterior major and minor, and sternocleidomastoid), and *muscles that help bow the head* (longus colli, sternocleidomastoid, scallenus anterior, medius and posterior, and rectus capitis).
The Action:	Neck extension, lateral flexion, rotation, and flexion.
Equipment You Need:	None.

The Workout:

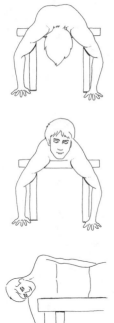
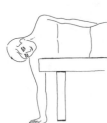
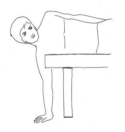

This workout is in *four* parts. Complete ten reps of Part One. Turn to one side for ten reps each of Parts Two and Three. Flip over to your other side and repeat Parts Two and Three. Then turn over on your back and complete Part Four.

PART ONE: Lie down on your abdomen on a bed or a table, and scoot over the edge until you are suspended out as far as your armpits. Dangle your arms straight down from your shoulders and brace yourself, if possible, by holding the legs of the bed or table with your hands, or by placing your palms on the floor. Relax your neck and drop your head. This is the starting position. Leading with your chin, curl your head up until you can go no farther. Resist the temptation to continue the neck curl into a back arch. Keep your back relaxed and out of the action. Hold for a moment. Return slowly to the starting position.

PART TWO: Turn over onto your side, and scoot over the edge until you are suspended out as far as your armpit. Keep your back straight. Dangle one arm straight down from your shoulder and brace yourself, if possible, by holding the leg of the bed or table with your hand, or by placing your palm on the floor. Place the other arm in line down the top side of your body. Tighten your abdominals to stabilize your position. Relax your neck and drop your head to the side. This is the starting position. Leading with your ear, curl your head up until you can go no farther. Hold for a moment. Return slowly to the starting position.

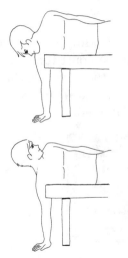

PART THREE: Stay on your side. Get your head in line with your spine. Your neck will be straight. This is the starting position. Rotate your neck so that you face the floor completely. Then rotate your neck so that you face the ceiling (or until you can go no farther). Hold for a moment. Return slowly to the starting position.

Remember: You've got a right and a left side! You have to flip over and do Parts Two and Three on the other side before you move to Part Four!

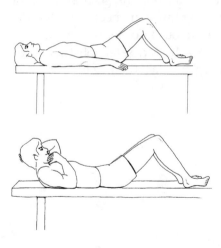

PART FOUR: Flip over onto your back and scoot down until your head is resting on the surface. Bend your knees and put your feet flat on the surface. Place one hand behind your head for a gentle assist at the end of the movement, and place the fingertips of the other hand on your chin to guide the tracking. Tuck your chin and lift your head until you can go no farther. When you are tucked and feel the muscles in the front and sides of your neck contract, assist with your hand by gently pressing your head forward, and then hold for a moment. The movement will be subtle and "crunchlike" rather than a head-up/head-down nod. Return slowly to the starting position.

Caution: This is an easy exercise to do incorrectly, because so many uninvited muscles—such as pectoralis muscles and deltoids—eagerly join in to help. You want to isolate your neck, giving it no choice but to do its own workout. Keep your mouth closed. We always have to remind Phil that incoming bugs are not part of an athlete's diet.

Managing Your Sets:

Ten reps of each of the four parts (including Parts Two and Three on both your left and right sides) constitutes one set. Transition from one exercise right into the next one. Because you will be alternating the four exercises, there is no need to rest between sets, unless you feel fatigued.

How long does it take when Jim and Phil work out?	
First Set:	2 minutes, 40 seconds
Second Set:	2 minutes, 40 seconds
Third Set:	2 minutes, 40 seconds
Total Time:	8 minutes

Taking It to the Gym:

In simple terms, you shouldn't. The weight of the average adult's head is approximately 7 to 11 pounds, so the weight of your head is adequate for working out your neck. Besides, the tissues in your neck are delicate. To our knowledge, no machine has been designed that will do a better, safer job than your own body. We recommend that you leave the machines alone.

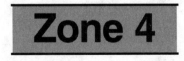

Zone 4

Arms, Elbows, Wrists, and Hands

27   Wrist Abductors and Adductors

What You Strengthen:	Muscles in the "thumb" sides of the forearms (flexor carpi radialis, and extensor carpi radialis longus and brevis), and muscles in the back of the forearms (flexor and extensor carpi ulnaris).
The Action:	Wrist abduction (radial flexion) and wrist adduction (ulnar flexion).
Equipment You Need:	One or two handheld weights (dumbbells).

The Workout:

This workout is in two parts.

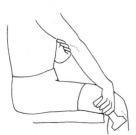

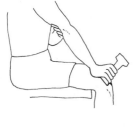

PART ONE: It really makes no difference whether you sit or stand, but we prefer standing. You can work both wrists at the same time, but when you do, remember to use equal weight on each side. With your arm straight down and your elbow locked, hold the weight in your hand with your palm facing in and your thumb forward. If you can, hold the weight at one end and extend the heavier part out to the *front*. Tuck your elbow tightly into your body between your hip bone and waist, so that you're stabilized and locked into position. If you're exercising only one arm at a time, the nonexercising arm should be relaxed, but you might feel more balanced and comfortable if you reach over with that arm and place your hand lightly on the front of the biceps at the elbow, to remind yourself to keep it straight. Start with the weight pointed down to the floor. Without bending your elbow, and using your hand and wrist, lift the weight straight up in front of you as far as possible. You'll feel the contraction in your forearm. Hold for a moment and then slowly lower the weight to the starting position. If you're working one wrist at a time, switch your weight to the other hand and complete ten reps. When you've completed ten reps on both sides (one at a time or both together), go to Part Two.

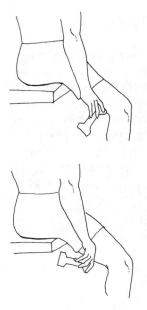

PART TWO: With your arm straight down and your elbow locked, hold the weight in your hand with your palm facing in and your thumb pointing forward. If you can, hold the weight at one end and extend the heavier part out to the *back*. Without bending your elbow, using your hand and wrist, lift the weight straight up in back of you as far as possible. You'll feel the contraction in the back of your forearm and on the outside of your elbow. Hold for a moment and then slowly lower the weight to the starting position. If you're working one wrist at a time, switch your weight to the other hand and complete ten reps.

Caution: It's really easy to let your fingers do all the work by flipping the weight up and supporting it on its way down. It might *look* like the same "lifting action," but we are not deceived. Hold that weight firmly. Make that wrist work.

Managing Your Sets:

Ten reps of each of the two parts (including both your left and right sides) constitute one set. Transition from one exercise right into the next one. Because you will be alternating the two exercises, there is no need to rest between sets, unless you feel fatigued.

How long does it take when Jim and Phil work out?	
First Set:	45 seconds
Second Set:	45 seconds
Third Set:	45 seconds
Total Time:	2 minutes, 15 seconds

Taking It to the Gym:

This is a free weight workout.

Zone 4

28 *Forearm Supinators and Pronators*

What You Strengthen:	The muscle that runs from the top of your upper arm, attaches below your elbow at the back of your forearm, and facilitates the unique rotating action of the forearm (biceps brachii); the muscle that runs from the top of the elbow at the humerus and the ridge of the ulna to wrap around and insert on the upper third of the radius (supinator); the muscle that attaches to the radius and ulna at the wrist (pronator quadratus); and the muscle that starts at the upper radius, wraps around the back (lateral) side of the bones, and ends at the mid-ulna (pronator teres).
The Action:	Wrist and forearm pronation and supination.
Equipment You Need:	One handheld weight (dumbbell).

The Workout:

This workout is in two parts.

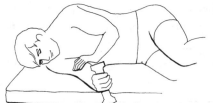

PART ONE: Lie on your side on a bed or table with your knees drawn up so that you are stabilized. Scoot over until your shoulder is at the edge of the surface, and align your upper arm so that it runs parallel with the edge. This is your exercising arm. Grip the weight in your hand with your palm forward and your thumb pointing *up*. If you have a choice, hold the weight at one end and allow the bulk of the weight to hang below your hand. Bend your elbow to position your forearm at a 90-degree angle to your upper arm and cantilever it out so that it's free from the surface and the weight "hangs" below your arm and hand. Remember: your thumb will be *up*. Use the hand of your nonexercising arm to stabilize your elbow by pressing very gently from above. Now pivot the weight up and over. Your thumb will now be *down*. Hold for a moment and then return slowly to the starting position.

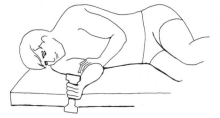

PART TWO: Now grip the weight in your hand with your palm backward and your thumb pointing *down*. If you have a choice, hold the weight at one end and allow the bulk of the weight to hang below your hand. Bend your elbow to position your forearm at a 90-degree angle to your upper arm, which should be parallel to the edge of the table. Cantilever it out so that it's free from the surface and the weight can "hang" below your arm and hand. Remember: your thumb will be *down*. Use the hand of your nonexercising arm to stabilize your elbow by pressing very gently from above. Now pivot the weight up and over. Your thumb will now be *up*. Hold for a moment and then return slowly to the starting position.

Managing Your Sets:

Complete ten reps of Part One with one hand and then, without changing sides, complete ten reps of Part Two. Change sides. When you have completed Part One and Part Two on BOTH sides, you have completed one set. Because you are alternating sides, there is no need to rest between sets, unless you feel fatigued.

How long does it take when Jim and Phil work out?	
First Set:	1 minute
Rest:	30 seconds
Second Set:	1 minute
Rest:	30 seconds
Third Set:	1 minute
Total Time:	4 minutes

Taking It to the Gym:

This is a free weight workout.

Zone 4

87

29 *Wrist Flexors and Extensors—The Roll-Up*

What You Strengthen:	Muscles in the inside (medial side) of the forearms (flexor carpi radialis, ulnaris, and palmaris longus) and muscles in the top (lateral side) of the forearms (extensor carpi radialis brevis and longus, and extensor carpi ulnaris).
The Action:	Both wrist flexion and extension. This is a carpal tunnel syndrome buster!
Equipment You Need:	Your own personal Wharton Roll-Up.

Before you can do this workout, you have to construct a piece of customized equipment. All you need is a dowel long enough for your hands to fit side-by-side with a knot of twine in between them, and thick enough so that you can comfortably grip it, or approximately one foot in length and one inch in diameter. For example, you could cut down a broom handle. (You can construct several Roll-Ups from a single handle. The added benefit is that the more you cut, the shorter the broom gets. When it's totally ruined, you have an excuse not to sweep. You'd rather work out anyway, right?) Next, cut a piece of twine the length of the distance between your waist and the floor. Tie one end to the middle of the dowel and secure it so that it doesn't slip. If you really want to get fancy, you can drill a hole through the dowel and knot the twine through it. Tie a light weight to the other end of the twine. Make sure the dowel is free from splinters and rough surfaces that will irritate your hands.

The Workout:

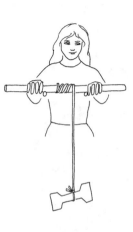

Stand with your back straight, your feet slightly apart, and your knees slightly bent. Let out all the twine on your Roll-Up so that the weight dangles as far from the dowel as possible. Your objective is to roll the twine onto the dowel by using a sort of "wringing action"—alternating your hands until the weight has been rolled up from the floor to the dowel. Hold the dowel in front of you with one hand on either side of the knot—palms down, thumbs facing each other. Straighten your arms and lock your elbows. You can position your arms at any angle to your body, as long as the dowel is parallel to the floor. The angle makes little difference, but the higher you hold the dowel, the greater will be the strain on your deltoids. First, loosen the grip of your left hand, roll it straight over the top to the front of the dowel, and regrip the dowel. Loosen your right hand, but don't let go. Roll the twine up by rolling the dowel back with your left hand. When you can go back no farther, "brake" it by gripping the dowel in your right hand. Then loosen the grip of your left hand and continue to roll the twine up by reaching over and rolling the dowel back with your right hand. Then left. Right. Left. Right. Continue until the twine is coiled tightly around the dowel between your hands and the weight is rolled all the way up. Then, let the weight down by using opposite action. Rolling it up and down by rotating the dowel toward you works your extensors. To work the opposite muscles—the flexors—repeat the roll up and down, but reverse the direction in which you rotate the dowel. In other words, roll your fists over the top. (In case you're wondering how fast to roll up and down, you might take a cue from Phil. He once got a whole class of adult athletic trainers to sing "Itsy Bitsy Spider" while they rolled. Admittedly, it was sort of annoying, but it *did* capture the rhythm of the action.)

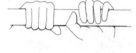
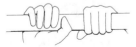

Managing Your Sets:

Start with the weight down toward the floor. Roll it back up to the dowel. When you've got it all the way up, roll it back down. This constitutes one set. Rest 30 seconds between sets.

How long does it take when Jim and Phil work out?	
First Set:	30 seconds
Rest:	*30 seconds*
Second Set:	30 seconds
Rest:	*30 seconds*
Third Set:	30 seconds
Total Time:	2 minutes, 30 seconds

Taking It to the Gym:

You can't (unless they'll let you bring your Roll-Up and sing "Itsy Bitsy Spider").

Zone 4

30 *Finger and Thumb Flexors*

What You Strengthen:	Hands and fingers (flexor digitorum profundus and superficialis, flexor pollicis longus and brevis, flexor carpi ulnaris, opponens pollicis, and flexor digiti minimi).
The Action:	Finger flexion (simply put, "grip").
Equipment You Need:	A foam ball, a foam pillow, or anything that you can get your fingers around that will spring back into shape after you squeeze it. If you want to get fancy, you can stuff the toe of a sock with tightly packed, shredded foam from a craft supply shop or sewing goods store.

Note: This workout is tailored to help relieve carpal tunnel syndrome and other repetitive stress injuries by strengthening muscles and releasing tension.

The Workout:

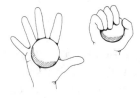

Hold the ball in the palm of your hand and slowly squeeze it until you can squeeze no more. Hold for a moment and then slowly release.

Managing Your Sets:

Rest thirty seconds between sets.

How long does it take when Jim and Phil work out?	
First Set:	15 seconds
Rest:	*10 seconds*
Second Set:	15 seconds
Rest:	*10 seconds*
Third Set:	15 seconds
Total Time:	1 minute, 5 seconds

Taking It to the Gym:

There are a lot of things you *could* squeeze at the gym, but the staff will probably discourage it. Do this workout at home.

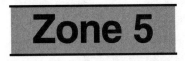

Zone 5

Lower Legs, Ankles, and Feet

31 Soleus

What You Strengthen:	Deep calf (soleus).
The Action:	Bent knee plantar flexion (extension).
Equipment You Need:	One or two handheld weights (dumbbells) or something with weight, such as a book.

The Workout:

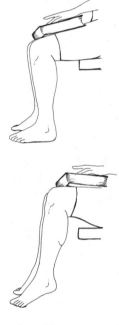

Sit on any surface that allows your thighs to be parallel to the floor, your knees to bend at 90-degree angles, and your feet to rest flat on the floor. Sit up straight and contract your abdominals to keep your torso stable. Put your knees and feet together. Place a weight across the top of your knees. (Remember to distribute the weight evenly between them.) This is the starting position. Roll up from the balls of your feet and toes to raise your heels straight up until you can go no farther. You'll feel contraction in your calves and pressure on the balls of your feet. Hold for a moment. Then slowly return to the starting position.

Caution: Your upper thighs might try to assist the action. Resist!

Managing Your Sets:

Ten reps constitute one set. Take a thirty-second rest between sets.

How long does it take when Jim and Phil work out?	
First Set:	40 seconds
Rest:	*30 seconds*
Second Set:	40 seconds
Rest:	*30 seconds*
Third Set:	40 seconds
Total Time:	3 minutes

Taking It to the Gym:

You can use any calf-raise machine that allows you to select your weight and, more important, to position your knees into 90-degree angles. Let us explain why the angles are specific and critical. When your knee is bent to 90 degrees, the outer calf muscle—the gastrocnemius—is disengaged at the upper attachment at the knee. When the gastrocnemius isn't involved, the soleus is forced to assume the lead role in raising and lowering your heel. It's allowed to do the work and get stronger. Also, on a machine, you should work out *one leg at a time.* When you work both simultaneously, the stronger one carries the load. It continues to get stronger while your weaker leg gets weaker. If the machine is designed to lock you into position to work both legs at the same time, simply relax one leg. Decrease the weight by 50 percent. It'll take you twice as long to complete the set, but you'll get an honest workout.

Note: The machines may tempt you to use too much weight. Use good judgment instead.

Zone 5

32 Gastrocnemius

What You Strengthen:	Calves (gastrocnemius or "gastrocs," and soleus), and arches of feet (plantaris).
The Action:	Straight knee plantar flexion (extension).
Equipment You Need:	A book that is two inches thick.

The Workout:

This exercise is done in three parts—not because the Whartons like to complicate things, but because the gastrocnemius is a complicated system. First, the muscle is split anatomically. It's considered to be one muscle, but in fact it arises from two distinct heads—the inside (medial) and the outside (lateral). Second, although it has two heads and the muscular masses are separate, it functions in perfect tandem as one muscle. The confusion continues even into its nomenclature. Although its proper name is gastrocnemius (singular), we nickname it the "gastrocs" (plural). Nicknames notwithstanding, we certainly do know how to train *all* of it (them?).

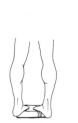

PART ONE: Find a book about two inches thick. Place it on the floor immediately in front of a table that you can use to stabilize your body. Facing the table, stand with your toes forward, the balls of your feet on the book, and your heels resting on the floor. This is the starting position. Place your hands on the table to balance. Raise your heels straight up until you're up on your toes as far as you can go. Then rock forward slightly and transfer some of your weight to your hands. By leaning on your hands, you get a little more height up on your toes and gain slightly more contraction in the gastrocs. When you can go no farther, hold for a moment and then lower your heels slowly to the starting position. This trains the medial and lateral arches and the entire back of the calf: the plantaris, the gastrocnemius, and the soleus. (These three muscles form a tripartite muscle mass that shares the Achilles or calcaneal tendon. Collectively, they are sometimes called the "triceps surae.")

PART TWO: Repeat the same action, but with your toes pointed *in* and your heels pointed *out* at 45-degree angles. This trains the inside (medial) aspect.

PART THREE: Repeat the same action, but with the toes pointed out and your heels pointed *in* at 45-degree angles. This trains the outside (lateral) aspect.

Note: Because of the weight of your body on these muscles, you begin your training by lifting both heels at the same time. Later, when you're more experienced, you can work one heel at a time to develop greater strength and balance.

Managing Your Sets:

Ten reps are done for each part. With a three-part workout, this means you have three sets, each consisting of three parts, with a rest in between each set.

How long does it take when Jim and Phil work out?	
First Set:	
Part One:	50 seconds
Part Two:	50 seconds
Part Three:	50 seconds
Rest:	*30 seconds*
Second Set:	
Part One:	50 seconds
Part Two:	50 seconds
Part Three:	50 seconds
Rest:	*30 seconds*
Third Set:	
Part One:	50 seconds
Part Two:	50 seconds
Part Three:	50 seconds
Total Time: 8 minutes,	30 seconds

Taking It to the Gym:

We prefer that you use a leg press. You'll get a full range of motion, and your feet will have direct contact with the force of the weight. Or, you can use a standing heel-raise machine, where you support weight at your shoulder as you raise and lower your heels. Avoid machines that require you to loop a wide belt around your waist and attach it to weight that you lift from your hips. This creates too much instability in your midsection. Increment weight and resistance very slowly.

33 Lower Leg Triple Play

What You Strengthen:	Lower leg (tibialis anterior and posterior, peroneus tertius, extensor hallucis longus, extensor digitorum longus, and peroneus brevis, tertius, and longus).
The Action:	Ankle dorsi flexion, and foot supination and pronation.
Equipment You Need:	A tube sock with a weight in the toe.

The Workout:

This workout is designed in two parts for two reasons. First, these muscles always function as a team. They work in concert to stabilize your feet and support your weight, keeping you upright and balanced. Second, when you're in position in the workout, it's efficient to continue from one exercise to the next.

Before you begin, you'll need to construct a piece of personal workout equipment. Take a long tube sock and stuff a one-pound weight down into the toe. If you don't have a weight, you may use anything that weighs a pound and is small enough to fit.

Tie the sock onto your exercising foot by dangling the weight under the ball of your foot and threading the sock between your big toe and the toe next to it ("second metatarsal" for those who enjoy technical accuracy, and "the piggy who stayed home" for all the rest of us). It doesn't matter how far down the weight hangs, but make certain that you have plenty of sock left to loop around your foot. Continue to wrap by looping the end of the sock around the outside of your foot, under your arch and back up over the top of your foot. Then fasten it securely by tying under the top wrap.

Note: You can work out both sides at the same time if you use two equally weighted socks.

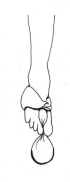

PART ONE: Sit on any surface that allows your thighs to be parallel to the floor, your knees to bend at a 90-degree angle, and your feet and sock-weights to dangle well above the floor. Sit up straight and contract your abdominals to keep your torso stable. You might want to place a rolled towel underneath your knees. This padding will take pressure off the kneecaps (patellae). Also, any time you sit with your knees slightly higher than your tail bone (coccyx), you reduce stress on your back. Slightly separate your knees and feet. Point your toes down straight to the floor. This is the starting position. Now, slowly raise the front of your foot until you can go no farther. Your heel will be down and your toes will be up. You'll feel contractions in the outside of your lower leg and the top of your foot. Hold for a moment and then slowly return to the starting position: toe pointed down.

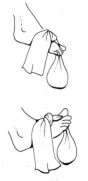

PART TWO: Maintain the same basic position, but this time point your toes straight down and come up by sweeping your foot to the inside and pointing your big toe to the ceiling. This is a diagonal movement. You'll feel contractions in your arch and in the inside of your lower leg. Sweep back down until your big toe is pointing straight to the floor. Hold for a moment. Then continue the sweep up and to the outside as far as you can go. Again, this is a diagonal movement. You'll feel contractions in the outside of your ankle and lower leg. Slowly return to the starting position: toe pointed down.

Managing Your Sets:

Ten reps of Parts One and Two combined constitute one set. There is no need to rest between sets, unless you feel fatigued.

How long does it take when Jim and Phil work out?	
First Set:	1 minute
Second Set:	1 minute
Third Set:	1 minute
Total Time:	3 minutes

Taking It to the Gym:

To our knowledge, there is no equipment that isolates the muscles as effectively as this simple exercise.

Zone 5

97

34 Ankle Evertors and Invertors

What You Strengthen:	Lower leg evertors (peroneus longus, brevis, and tertius, and extensor digitorum longus) and lower leg invertors (tibialis anterior and posterior, and extensor hallucis longus).
The Action:	Foot and ankle eversion and inversion.
Equipment You Need:	One or two ankle weights.

The Workout:

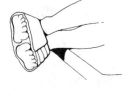

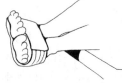

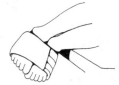

This workout exercises evertors and invertors simultaneously. You're going to exercise both ankles at the same time.

Lie on your side on a table or bed. Wrap the ankle weights under the arches and over the top of both feet. Straighten your legs and lock your knees. Hang your feet over the edge. Relax them, allowing them to drop into neutral positions. Contract your abdominals to stabilize your position and protect your back. This is your starting position. Rotate both feet up toward you, as if you are trying to point the bottom of your feet toward the ceiling. When you can go no farther, hold for a moment. On the top leg, you will feel contractions from the outside of your lower leg to your ankle. This is eversion. On the lower leg, you'll feel contractions from the inside of your lower leg to your arch. This is inversion. Return to the starting position.

When you have completed three sets on one side, flip over and complete three sets on the other side.

Managing Your Sets:

When you have completed ten reps working both left and right ankles, this constitutes one set. Rest thirty seconds between sets.

How long does it take when Jim and Phil work out?		
First Set:	1 minute	
Rest:		*30 seconds*
Second Set:	1 minute	
Rest:		*30 seconds*
Third Set:	1 minute	
Total Time:	3 minutes	

Taking It to the Gym:

To our knowledge, there is no equipment that isolates the muscles as effectively as this simple exercise.

35 Feet Arches

What You Strengthen:	Medial arch of foot (plantaris, adductor hallucis, tibialis posterior, peroneus longus brevis, flexor hallucis longus and brevis, supinators, and pronators).
The Action:	Arching and flattening the arch.
Equipment You Need:	A towel. Later, when you have more experience, you might want to add a weight.

The Workout:

This exercise is done in three parts. Once you're in position, it's efficient to move from one action to the next.

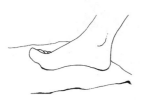

PART ONE: For this workout, you need to have a floor surface on which a towel will slide easily. First, position a towel on the floor straight out in front of a chair. Sit in the chair with your back straight and your bare feet flat on the edge of the towel. This is the start position. Work only one foot at a time. Without moving your heel, contract all your toes to bunch up the towel and gather it toward you until you have done ten repetitions (bunches) or run out of towel. This strengthens your medial arch for propulsion and your lateral arch for bearing weight.

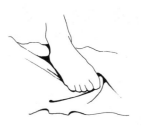

PART TWO: Straighten out the towel and turn it sideways. Keep your heel on the towel. Starting with your little toe, contract all your toes to bunch up the towel tightly and sweep it toward the midline of your body. The mental imagery we use is that you're bringing your *little* toe under your foot to meet your *big* toe, and you're going under the floor to do it. It's an under-the-floor "U." Without moving your heel, continue to gather and sweep the towel until you have done ten repetitions or run out of towel. This strengthens your supinators.

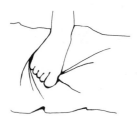

PART THREE: Straighten out the towel, but leave it sideways. Keep your heel on the towel. Starting with your big toe, contract all your toes to bunch up the towel tightly and sweep it away from the midline of your body. The mental imagery we use is that you're bringing your *big* toe under your foot to meet your *little* toe, and you're going under the floor to do it. It's an under-the-floor "U." Without moving your heel, continue to gather and sweep the towel until you have done ten repetitions or run out of towel. This strengthens your pronators.

Note: As you get stronger, you might want to place a weight at the far end of the towel. It makes the bunching more difficult as you drag the weight across the floor.

Managing Your Sets:

It's easier to work one foot at a time and take it through an entire set. One combination of all three parts on one foot constitutes one set. There is no need to rest between sets, unless you feel fatigued.

How long does it take when Jim and Phil work out?		
First Set	(Right):	1 minute
	(Left):	1 minute
Second Set	(Right):	1 minute
	(Left):	1 minute
Third Set	(Right):	1 minute
	(Left):	1 minute
Total Time:	6 minutes	

Taking It to the Gym:

To our knowledge, there is no equipment that isolates the muscles as effectively as this simple exercise.

Part III

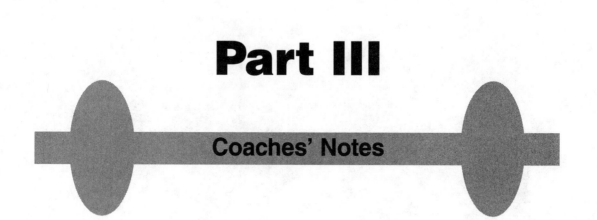

Coaches' Notes

O K, Athlete! It's time to put the program together. To decide which strengthening exercises you need to help you build a winner's body, you need only run through the Coaches' Notes and identify all the sports and occupational activities you do every day, or are planning to make part of your life. Remember that any time you use your body to accomplish a task, you're an athlete who deserves an athlete's advantages in training and performance. Once you make that connection, you'll find yourself making major strides in your everyday activities, in your sports, and on the job.

If you decide to train for an upcoming sport, or your activities change with the seasons, you have information at hand that will help you adjust your workouts to meet the new demands. In thumbing through the Coaches' Notes, you might even spot a new activity that sounds like fun and decide to give it a try. Almost everyone earmarks several that are intriguing.

At the start of the Coaches' Notes for each activity, we catalog the zones of the body that either benefit from additional specific strength work, or are completely left out of the activity and need to be taken care of. Additionally, we've given you the numbers of the relevant exercises described and pictured in Part II.

The zones are:

Zone 1   **Upper Legs, Hips, and Trunk (The Foundation)**

Zone 2   **Shoulders**

Zone 3   **Neck**

Zone 4   **Arms, Elbows, Wrists, and Hands**

Zone 5   **Lower Legs, Ankles, and Feet**

As you list your own activities and make notes on the exercises you'll need, you'll inevitably discover overlaps. No problem. And no need to do anything twice. Just mesh the workouts and develop a single program.

Within the text of the Coaches' Notes, we give you anecdotes, tips, and advice that we have gleaned from years of experience and research. It's the same discussion we have with our professional athletes who are beginning a training or rehab program.

Enjoy!

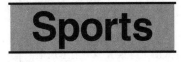

Sports

Baseball/Softball

To Strengthen:	Upper Legs, Hips, and Trunk	1–15
	Shoulders	16–25
	Neck	26
	Arms, Elbows, Wrists, and Hands	27–30
	Lower Legs, Ankles, and Feet	31–35

Coaches' Notes

In sports circles, a debate rages over whether American baseball was an evolution of British cricket or a revolution against it. Probably a little of both. Baseball as we know it took flight in the late 1850s when Harry Wright, a cricket champion, joyfully joined the New York Knickerbockers baseball team and ushered his newly favorite game into the realms of professional sports. The *Cincinnati Enquirer* described Wright as a man who "eats base-ball, breathes base-ball, thinks base-ball, dreams base-ball, and incorporates base-ball into his prayers." His personal obsession developed into a great all-American sport—and a great all-American obsession.

If you evaluate the relative danger of a sport based on the amount of protective gear and clothing that accompanies a player onto the field, then baseball looks relatively safe. No suits of armor. Not much padding. Helmet only when batting. But looks can be deceiving. Baseball is second only to football in total number of injuries and fatalities. Why the apparent contradiction? Because, baseball has so many participants that the sheer numbers overwhelm the statistical percentages. In other words, lots of people get hurt, but your chances of being one of them are slim.

One of the real challenges in analyzing the biomechanics of baseball is that the sport involves intricate relationships between function and coordination. Truly, if there's one sport where "May The Force Be With You" applies, this is it. If you doubt it for a second, think about pitching. Your entire body winds up in a tight torque with one foot off the ground. You look away from the batter for a second. You make the decision that all systems are on "go." You unwind explosively, transmit that energy, and fire the ball with precise speed, force, spin, and direction. You continue to unwind your torqued position until you regain perfect balance. Then you return your body to a "ready" posture in case you need to field a ball being hit back to you. All this takes place in a split second and requires perfect focus and coordination.

We chose the repetitious, high-velocity pitch to represent the intricacies of baseball because the pitch is the source of most injuries. Shoulders, arms, wrists, and hands are the injured sites we most commonly see. And, if you think that side-arm pitching is safer, think again. Statistics verify that the injury rate is identical to that of the traditional hardball throw. The shoulder—no matter how you pitch—is particularly vulnerable because of the enormous stress placed on it. Although it's true that the shoulder is functionally highly mobile and allows the arm to move in all directions, it is surprisingly fragile. In the truest definition of a "joint," the shoulder joins parts of the body (the arms to the torso), but it is neither highly muscled nor vascularized itself. Instability and weakness are not uncommon. In strengthening the shoulder, you have to work the body on both sides of the joint, because the shoulder's strength and stability are direct results of the collective strength and stability of the anatomical areas it joins.

But the shoulder isn't the only area that needs to be protected in baseball, and danger is not limited to pitching. Experts note that impact injuries of the head and neck constitute half the fatalities. Collisions with bases, balls, bats, and other players put baseball players at real risk. Another culprit is sliding—where a movable force (the face of a player hurtling horizontally) meets an immovable object (the baseman's foot). And there's more. Even a quietly squatting, seemingly safe catcher is subject to a litany of injuries that include hand injuries (from repetitive smacking of a ball against the palm and fingers), knee problems from squatting, and collisions with out-of-control runners, balls, bats, and evil-tempered managers. Finally, there is the problem of explosive running—going from 0 to 60 in a split second, with no opportunity for warming up. (If the score is tied, the other team is at bat, and you see a fly ball rocketing toward you, you aren't going to stop to stretch and do a few arm swings before you dive for the catch.)

Weight training is essential to build balance, stability, and endurance, particularly in the shoulder. And remember that success absolutely depends on working the anatomical areas that surround the shoulders—front, back, top, and bottom. In addition, as a baseball player, you are also a sprinter. You need leg strength to power home runs, to stretch a double into a triple, and to chase the would-be hits of the opposing team.

A final note: Success in baseball demands that you warm up before you play. Equally important and doubly difficult, you have to stay warmed up for the duration of the game. This may require that you stay in constant motion during play, whether you're on the field or in the dugout.

Basketball

Coaches' Notes

We usually meet an athlete in our clinic after he or she is already racked up and has faced the very real possibility that the career built on sports or dance is about to give way to watching other people do it on television. One of the few exceptions to this client-pattern is basketball players. We see them when they are healthy, in top form, and still trying to get even better. Our experience is echoed by sports medicine researchers who agree that almost all basketball players are naturally endowed with superior neuromuscular control and, thanks to the demands of their game, are in great shape. Frankly, you can't play the game unless you are a gifted athlete in great shape. Anything less and your jersey number might as well be 911.

Because the players come to the court with a double dose of good genes and hard work, injuries in basketball are relatively few. Most frequently, those that occur are caused by trauma. (The same could be said of the fans; but that's a different kind of trauma, isn't it?) We see a lot of cuts and bruises caused by collision. The more serious the impact, the more serious the injury can be, so we can expand our list of basketball injuries to include sprains, strains, and fractures. When we speak of impact, we mean the head-on crunch of player to player or player to sportscaster table, but we also mean the pounding of the foot on the floor as a single player runs and jumps. Logically, the injuries start with the foot (where the rubber-soled shoe meets the urethaned-hardwood floor) and work their way up through the ankle, knee, and hip.

The benefits of fitness in preventing injury go without saying (but we'll do it anyway). The more generally fit you are, the more you are able to dodge an out-of-control player who's careening across the court with you in his path. Or better yet, you can prevent being an out-of-control player yourself. Being in control has more value than merely preventing collision. It means that you can put your body and the ball where you intend them to be.

Because most injuries start with the foot, it stands to reason that your feet deserve extra attention in training. We want to caution you about two things: first, just because you're playing in high-topped basketball shoes, you can't assume that you have any sort of ankle support; and second, taping healthy ankles as a matter of routine restricts movement, creates chronic weakness, and gives you a false sense of security. Your foot is a remarkable shock absorber. It was designed to work in a system with your ankle, knee, and hip to allow you to move in any direction, to change that direction, to spring, and to land. Any imbalance, weakness, or flaw in the system will set off a chain reaction of compensations as your body valiantly attempts to adjust itself to get the job done. It starts at the floor. If your feet can't absorb shock because the muscles are weak, then your ankles take up the slack. If your ankles can't hold the position, your knees adjust and give assistance. If your knees can't handle it, your hips take the hit. If your hips fail, your back locks in. Before you know it, you're in real trouble.

Experts pass along two noteworthy tips: (1) Warm up before you step on the court, and (2) try to sit out a play when you're tired. Playing when you're ill-prepared for the activity or when you're too fatigued to be in control are two major contributors to serious injury (and abysmal scores).

Part of the excitement of basketball is the second-by-second, unexpected unfolding of strategies by both teams. To be a great player, you have to be prepared for anything at any time. You might have a skill that's your trademark specialty, but you have to be a generalist. For this reason, practicing every skill and achieving overall conditioning are critical. We want you to look good for all your endorsement deals, and we want you to play even better.

Bodybuilding

To Strengthen:	Upper Legs, Hips, and Trunk	1–15
	Shoulders	16–25
	Arms, Elbows, Wrists, and Hands	27–30
	Lower Legs, Ankles, and Feet	31–35

Coaches' Notes

When we met our first bodybuilder, we had a difficult time grasping the concept of weight lifting as an end rather than a means. It seemed to be training for a sport one would never play. Later, as our familiarity with the practice grew with experience, we began to regard bodybuilding as an amalgam of sport and art—literally, sculpture. The training IS the sport. And the result is a body that is painstakingly shaped with time and sweat.

In the past decade, we have witnessed a revolution in bodybuilding as it has emerged into the mainstream. Bodybuilding was once the mysterious domain of the seriously obsessed. The vocabulary reeked of bloodshed. "He's buff. She's cut. They're ripped." The bodybuilders were suspiciously tanned (even in the dead of winter in Milwaukee) and basted in oil. And there was talk of drugs that turned up the volume on testosterone for men and women, and magically grew huge muscles in all the right places and hair in all the wrong ones. But the worst of early bodybuilding was the misinformation that was passed from lifter to lifter in locker rooms all over the world. The field was rife with super-stition and a frenzied quest for potions, powders, and pills that would pump up, pop out, and press down body parts. It was dangerous. And people paid for it with their health. Some died.

Today, sports medicine and research have supplanted the mythol-ogy that once threatened to lead well-intentioned bodybuilders into self-destruction. The gyms have moved solidly into the information age. The governing bodies of the sport have imposed strict sanctions that prohibit the use of deadly chemistry. And the trainers are now cer-tified, licensed, educated, and more experienced than at any other time in history. The result is a reformed sport that now deserves a measure of respect. Bodybuilders are legitimate athletes.

Now that we've said all the nice stuff, let us say that bodybuilders are notorious for looking fit, but falling short in aerobic endurance. It's true that, compared to sedentary individuals, bodybuilders' aerobic ca-pacity (maximum oxygen consumption) may increase a small to mod-erate amount with high-volume weight training, but it is nowhere near the level it should be. Increasing that capacity is a bit of problem be-cause if you jog or ride a stationary bike hard enough to put your body into an anaerobic state, you compromise your ability to lift. There is a way, however. If you use increased high-volume lifting or interval training (hard-hard-easy, hard-hard-easy), your power to lift will be unimpeded while you increase your oxygen-carrying capacity.

Overuse injuries in bodybuilding are common and are often the result of overtraining. If you're obsessed by this sport—and you have to be in order to body-build—you will not understand this concept. Trust us. It's entirely possible to train too hard or too long. The problem with an overuse injury is that it leads to other difficulties such as muscle im-balances in the group opposite the injured site, a deterioration or com-pensation in your form and technique, and tightening of the tissue around the injury to protect it.

Injuries should be treated on a case-by-case basis by an expert who understands the concept of "active rest." If your doc says, "If it hurts, quit doing it," then you may assume that he or she is familiar with the physiology of an athlete, but not the drive. Stifle the urge to laugh out loud, but do leave skid marks on your way out the door. Find a professional who can design your rehabilitation without plunging you into total body atrophy. And when you find that professional, pay attention. Investment in proper, intelligent, patient rehabilitation yields huge dividends later. Look upon rehab as an opportunity to learn more about anatomy and to explore other aspects of your sport.

Caution: A special word to female bodybuilders: Nature deposits a layer of fat around the muscles of all women, masking to some extent the development and definition you work so hard to achieve. Dieting to lower your fat content can help solve this pesky problem. But dropping your percentage of body fat below 16 percent may cause your estrogen levels to diminish, possibly resulting in your losing estrogen's cardioprotective properties, developing amenorrhea, and running an increased risk of osteoporosis. Every woman is different, so you and your physician will want to monitor your body carefully and make intelligent decisions that take into consideration the long-term consequences of dieting.

Bowling

To Strengthen:	Upper Legs, Hips, and Trunk	1–15
	Shoulders	16–25
	Arms, Elbows, Wrists, and Hands	27–30

Coaches' Notes

Karen came to us with one request: "Make me rough and tough." We quickly agreed, "OK. Which sport?" We salivated with anticipation. Phil sat forward in his chair with his eyes flashing. The man loves a challenge. Karen replied, "Bowling." Phil sat back. But we were off on a biomechanical adventure that only a Wharton can know.

It was a little difficult to explore the literature on bowling because, frankly, it's not one of the games that attracts high-profile physiological research. We decided to take to the field and see for ourselves what makes bowling the number one participation sport in the United States (54 million bowlers!). We were pleasantly surprised when we walked into a bowling alley and found people of all ages and persuasions having a great time together. At once we decided that bowling is a joyful pursuit for anyone interested in fun, camaraderie, safety, and silly shoes.

Let us tell you what you already know. Bowling is not great exercise. Studies recently published by Florida State University indicate that bowling is SOME exercise (more than previously suspected). But we're here to tell you that it's not great. Sorry. That's the bad news.

The good news is that the injury rate on bowling is practically nonexistent. In fact, apparently the only documented injury exclusively associated with bowling is nerve damage to the thumb (perineural fibrosis of the ulnar digital nerve, or "Bowler's Thumb"). The cause? Ball hole is too small. Rehab for the bowler? None. Rehab for the ball? Drill a bigger hole.

More good news is that if you're like Karen and decide to train for the game like an athlete, you're likely to get better at it. And you will certainly get more fit. The stronger your body is, the heavier the ball you can lift and the more control you have over speed and spin on it as you release it. Additionally, we couldn't help but notice that nearly everyone was wearing wrist guards. As we told Karen, wrist guards indicate weakness. And weakness is vulnerability in any athlete. As Karen's training progressed and she felt comfortable, she was able to bowl without the brace. In discarding it, two things happened: Karen's wrist was allowed full range of motion so she could get even stronger and more balanced. And, equally important, her competitors were intimidated by this act of newfound bravado.

Our advice to bowlers: Enjoy your game, but supplement your fitness with a program that addresses physical activity with strength, flexibility, cardiovascular fitness, and endurance.

Boxing

To Strengthen:	Upper Legs, Hips, and Trunk	1–15
	Shoulders	16–25
	Neck	26
	Arms, Elbows, Wrists, and Hands	27–30
	Lower Legs, Ankles, and Feet	31–35

Coaches' Notes

As professionals who coach athletes to train their bodies to maximum performance levels, we are naturally confused by boxing, where injury is deliberately inflicted and damage is not only the result, but indeed the goal. The medical risks are catastrophic, so we will not recommend boxing as a sport of choice. We will, however, tell you that *training* for boxing is a fabulous way to get into shape. Please note that we make a clear distinction between *training* for boxing and actually boxing. Some of the most effective personal trainers we know are retired boxing coaches.

A couple of years ago, one of our flexibility clients invited us to join him for a workout session with his new fitness trainer. Excitedly, he told us that the trainer was one of these retired boxing coaches. In fact, this guy is so famous that we recognized his name and those of his boxers instantly. But, rather than share our client's excitement at his inclusion in the company of giants, we approached the invitation with trepidation and dread. We had visions of arriving at the gym just behind the ambulance, one step ahead of the helicopter medevac, and right beside the lawyers. In fact, Jim got out our client's medical records and placed them in the front of the file. "Just in case," he remarked grimly. When we arrived at the gym, we found our client darting up and down the indoor basketball court, shooting baskets with the boxing coach. Instead of a broken nose, we found a fast break in progress. It was a pleasant surprise. We were soon to learn that training for boxing employs all sorts of methods and can be a highly effective way to get into shape (without getting pounded into scrambled tofu).

Training for boxing combines the best of cardiovascular work with strength and coordination. As a sport that's centered around punching, it places heavy demands on the upper body: back, arms, and shoulders. At the same time, the constant dancing works out the lower body: legs and hips. To meet the demands of endurance, fighters include a cardio program. The net effect is a comprehensive, well-rounded workout regimen.

In addition to applauding the physical benefits of the sport, enthusiasts cite the mental and emotional extras. Pounding a bag helps release natural aggression and frustration that might otherwise surface at inappropriate moments and in unattractive ways—for example, at staff meetings where the temptation to leap across the conference table and pulverize your boss might be overwhelming.

A word of warning about trying to make weight: Don't. Doing crazy things like sweating in a sauna WILL allow an athlete to drop a few pounds, but he or she also runs the risk of cardiac function disturbances, heat stroke, and acutely impaired renal function. Not only is performance threatened; life is on the line. It takes up to 48 hours to replenish glycogen stores in the muscles, and 24 to 36 hours to recover from dehydration. Frankly, between the final weigh-in and the match, there isn't time to bring the body back to 100 percent. We join the American Medical Association and the American College of Sports Medicine in their condemnation of this practice. If you think you're weighing in as too heavy, check the scales. In 1948, at the Olympic Games, Bantam Weight Arnoldo Pares of Argentina weighed in as too heavy. His team panicked, cut off his hair, rubbed him down with a towel, scrubbed the dead skin and calluses off the bottom of his feet, and blew the dust off the scales. Pares even cried for a few minutes. It was futile. He couldn't make weight. The Argentine team filed a protest, forcing the Olympic Committee to summon an expert on weights and measures. Good thing. The scales were off. Pares, bald and with soft feet, cleared his weight and was allowed to box.

If you are going to spar, you MUST wear all the protective equipment available to you. If none is available, take off the gloves and step out of the ring. Yo, Adrian!

Canoeing

To Strengthen:	Upper Legs, Hips, and Trunk	1–15
	Shoulders	16–25
	Arms, Elbows, Wrists, and Hands	27–30

Coaches' Notes

Naturalist Henry David Thoreau said, "Everyone must believe in something. I believe I'll go canoeing." We think you should join him. Canoeing can be approached on many levels and is therefore available to people of all ages and in all kinds of shape. At one end of the canoeing spectrum, we have the young lovers drifting across a glassy lake: a smitten lad serenading with a ukulele, and his rosy gal reclining under her parasol while she falls in love. At the other end of the spectrum, we have the Olympic competitor who long ago traded the ukulele for adrenaline and a bone-jarring, teeth-gritting, nerve-shattering Class V rapid. Most of us fall somewhere in the middle of the two extremes. The point is that a canoe and paddle can be molded into a personal adventure and tailored workout of your own choosing.

Using a canoe for your workout requires that you make a decision about time and intensity. You have three choices. You can choose an anaerobic workout (paddle hard for a short time). You can choose an aerobic workout (paddle easily for a long time). Or you can choose an interval (tempo) workout (alternating paddling hard and easily).

Needless to say, paddling a canoe works the upper body—arms, shoulders, trunk, and back—to power your action and balance your body as you pivot and lean. But, because you are sitting or kneeling, your legs are used primarily to brace. Not only is range of motion limited, but opportunity to use muscles is restricted. The outcome is a serious disparity in muscular balance, strength, and flexibility. From the hips up, you are likely to be exceedingly well muscled. But from the hips down, you run the risk of being weak and underdeveloped. And your cardiovascular capacity might be woeful. For an athlete, it's an inexcusable combination. And it's also why most serious paddlers incorporate a good aerobic workout—running, cycling, or swimming—into their programs and spend extra time at the gym strengthening their legs and hips with weights.

Because paddling is repetitive motion and because a canoeist sits in one basic position for hours, he or she runs the risk of an injury one of our clients sarcastically calls "carpal tunnel body." As witty as our client is, overuse injuries are no laughing matter. Canoeists should be wary of nerve impingements, pain, numbness, and severe fatigue in hands, wrists, arms, and shoulders. Muscle cramps in the back and hips will take all the fun out of paddling. We suggest that you condition your body so that every muscle is able to do its job without fatiguing and having to recruit help from other muscles that will subsequently also fatigue and cramp. And we suggest that you change positions as frequently as you are able—even if it means merely shifting in your seat to take the pressure off your fanny for a moment. Move and stretch your legs once in a while. Most of all, have a good time. This is what canoes are all about.

Cricket

To Strengthen:	Upper Legs, Hips, and Trunk	1–15
	Shoulders	16–25
	Neck	26
	Arms, Elbows, Wrists, and Hands	27–30
	Lower Legs, Ankles, and Feet	31–35

Coaches' Notes

Years ago, we were invited to work with a cricket team just outside of London. As Americans, our knowledge of the intricacies of the sport was fairly limited, so we planted ourselves front-row-center to study the game and the athletes we were being asked to evaluate. Our first observation was that some of the players appeared to be slightly overweight—an unexpected and confusing contradiction to the obvious aerobic demands of the sport. And we also determined that cricket must be a genteel game played by genteel ladies and gentlemen. (After all, they *were* all wearing white.) We were wrong on both counts. Later, in the locker room, we discovered that the apparent overweight is in fact padding: a full chest protector that looks like a bulletproof vest, thigh pads (a larger one on the leading leg), forearm guards, gloves, an athletic cup, and leg guards that run from the top of the feet to just above the knees. The ensemble is topped by a helmet with a face visor. The reason for armor that would rival the swaddling of an NYPD swat team? Cricket is anything but genteel. It is, in fact, a dynamic, lightning fast-paced sport with some decidedly aggressive strategies. For example, in one play (a "bouncer"), a bowler bounces the ball toward the head and trunk of a batsman, who is expected to fend it off without suffering injury or emotional trauma. And did we mention that the ball can reach speeds of 90 mph? So much for the white uniforms and the grand illusions of gentility.

Injuries are specific to the activities involved with cricket. Bowling—propelling the ball—is more akin to the javelin toss than to pitching in American baseball. And the injuries are nearly identical. Lower spine strain is common as the bowler runs up, arches his back, rotates his hips, and then swings into and through the bowl. And the required straight elbow (distinguishing a bowl from a "throw") strains the shoulder—specifically, the rotator cuff. Nerve impingement and overuse injuries are the most common in the sport. In fielding, we tend to see injuries associated with quietly waiting for action and then ballistically springing into action. Muscles are cold. Players are tense. The ball rockets into the field. Reaction is split-second and dynamic. Something tears. And the cricketer finds himself in a bit of a "sticky wicket." It happens all the time.

Being fit goes a long way in maximizing performance levels, preventing injury, and winning. The good news is that cricket players are in better shape today than in any other time in history. The popularity of one-day play has placed greater physical demands on the players, who must rely on stamina, strength, speed, and flexibility to survive the rigors of the accelerated game. Additionally, the game is popular with players who are growing older—and wiser. Indeed, if you want to continue to play through your middle years and later, you had better be in good shape. And finally, the technologies of sports medicine have found their way into cricket. Training and rehabilitation methods have never been better. As in all ball sports, the foundation for success is a great fitness program that builds a strong player who can run.

Cross-Country Skiing

To Strengthen:	Upper Legs, Hips, and Trunk	1–15
	Shoulders	16–25
	Arms, Elbows, Wrists, and Hands	27–30
	Lower Legs, Ankles, and Feet	31–35

Coaches' Notes

Cross-country skiing is the ultimate cross-training sport. Cross our hearts. It places great stress on the cardiovascular system and, when done right, fires nearly every muscle in your body. Consequently, it is a fabulous workout. Not only that, but it gets you out in the fresh air and sunshine during a season of the year when many athletes wrap themselves in blankets, pour cups of hot cocoa, press themselves against frosted windows, and mourn the off-season. Not so with a cross-country skier.

Until recent years, it was impossible to study injuries in cross-country skiers, because medical researchers were not able to identify and track them. Quite literally, they are scattered everywhere. Downhill skiers cluster at mountains with ski lifts. Ski jumpers cluster at mountains with jumps. But cross-country skiers slide out their front doors and hit the trail, whether or not a trail exists. Consequently, identifying the difficulties and designing training and rehab methods have been slower than in other sports. Or less necessary. (By the way, we once skied right down the middle of Central Park West when a blizzard barricaded all the taxis in their garages and turned New York City into a deserted winter wonderland.)

Injuries, when they do occasionally occur, seem to center around trauma—accidents that happen when a skier using lightweight equipment reaches high speed, loses control, and falls or hits something. Studies also suggest that overuse or repetitive injuries of the shin, Achilles tendon, ankle, knee, and lower back are common. In fact, they might comprise 50 percent of all injuries that force skiers to lay off the sport for a significant period of healing.

Experts agree that injury prevention is less a matter of physical conditioning than of learning how to select trails that are safe and free from potential hazards. Failing that, a cross-country skier should know how to fall without getting hurt. (Phil practices this all the time.)

One of the interesting things about cross-country skiing is that it's an outdoor sport that can be brought indoors. (Don't try this with downhill or jumping!) There are a number of good ski-track machines on the market that simulate the action of cross-country skiing. The one we have in our clinic is a big favorite of clients who want quick, effective cardiovascular workouts, and of athletes with injuries that preclude impact to feet, legs, and hips. Lock your feet into narrow, sliding, parallel rails; turn on the CD player; slip on your heart monitor, set your timer, calibrate your resistance, grasp the handles of the arm pulleys, shout "Mush, you huskies!" and take off. The machines are inexpensive, quiet, lightweight, easily stored, and highly effective.

Technique notwithstanding, cross-country skiing, like all sports, is more fun when you are strong and flexible, and have the cardiovascular endurance to enjoy yourself. But, if you are not fit when you begin, check with a doctor and take heart. You'll be fit in short order (if you don't follow Jim into a pine tree).

Cycling

Coaches' Notes

A few years ago, Trevor McDonald limped into our clinic with one of the most unusual cycling injuries we had ever seen. Evaluation revealed that he was suffering with an unfortunate malady of inexperienced cyclists or cyclists who "up" their mileage without proper preparation. He had nerve compression syndrome in both of his hands and in his crotch. The symptoms were frightening numbness and lack of function. The syndrome in the hands is caused by unrelenting weight and pressure from leaning onto handle grips. The syndrome in the crotch is from sitting too long on a seat that is too hard and does not conform to human anatomy as we know it. Both injuries are seriously uncomfortable. How did this happen? Trevor whispered, "Tour de France." We were impressed, but we also knew that the Tour was not yet completed. If Trevor had been injured on the Tour, he should have been in the Alps and not in our clinic in New York. And further, we knew that no one on that professional level would make biomechanical mistakes with consequences of this magnitude. We gently struggled with contradictions in logic as we asked to see Trevor's bike so that we could examine the offending handle grips and seat. Trevor reluctantly admitted that he didn't actually own a bike. Our inquiry took a decided left turn. "OK, fella. How did you do all this damage in the Tour de France if you obviously weren't there and you have no bicycle?" The bizarre story unfolded as we sat, amazed. Trevor is an accountant who never left Manhattan. In fact, he never left his apartment. He had a stationary bike in his living room. He was participating in a "virtual" Tour de France ride with people he met on the Internet. They all cycled the exact distances on the exact days (or nights, after work) as the real riders on the Tour. The problem was that Trevor had not trained. And now, with these injuries, we could assure him that he wasn't going to win the cyber-jersey that day. But he was going to get a great education in anatomy and physiology. (And we will end the suspense and tell you that he's doing fine. Trevor eventually bought a real bicycle and actually went outside with it.)

In truth, cycling can be an invaluable cardiovascular component in a comprehensive fitness program. In fact, it can provide the stellar benefits of running without the impact on feet, legs, and hips. But there are a few ground rules for entering the sport. First, consult an expert when you're making a decision about what kind of bike to purchase. Second, take an expert with you to make certain that the bike is fitted to your body and outfitted to suit your needs. Third, realize that buying the bike isn't the end of your responsibility. The bike will require maintenance, safety checks, and adjustments throughout your relationship. Either learn to do these things yourself or align yourself with an experienced professional who can do them for you. And finally, learn how to ride. Know how to position your body and learn how to handle the bike. Work up slowly in intensity, distance, and duration. And train for cycling like you would any other sport.

Injuries in cycling are many and varied. Trauma—getting thrown from the bike onto the pavement—is the most common. Wearing protective gear, staying alert when riding, and maintaining a superior level of fitness will mitigate the potential for accidents, but, sadly, they are a fact of life when you cycle. What CAN be prevented, however, are overuse injuries (like Trevor's) caused by locking the body into the fanny-up/head-forward position, and pedaling with bent knees in a limited range of motion. Nerve impingement, muscular weakness, and imbalance are painful and debilitating, and can cause other serious problems. In addition, sudden increases in load, such as when sprinting and climbing hills, can place unusual strain on muscles and tendons. The list of injuries associated with cycling is as long as it is disturbing. The answer to all your potential problems is intelligence. Think. Realize that your body is locked into an unnatural position and that you're not allowing any joint to flex or extend through full ranges of motion. Compensate. Add strength work to your training program, to work muscles you're not firing at all on the bike, and to work muscles you are firing, but not fully. Add a flexibility program to your workout, to counteract the weaknesses caused by limited ranges of motion.

A final note: Please remember to hydrate when you ride. Cyclists sometimes forget how much they are sweating and need to replenish fluids. As they rocket along the road, air passes over their bodies, evaporating the sweat and cooling the skin. They're riding in a constant breeze that automatically adjusts itself to their speed. They ride slowly and experience a gentle breeze. They ride fast and experience a gale force wind. The problem is that cyclists may be deceived into thinking that cool and comfortable skin equals a cool and comfortable core temperature. Wrong. Heat problems set in when dehydration lowers the circulating volume of blood and the body's core temperature starts to rise. Problems manifest themselves in symptoms that include fatigue, lack of coordination, muscle pain and cramping, headache, lightheadedness, confusion, disorientation, and fainting. Under extreme circumstances, death can occur. Dehydration is a serious problem. If you feel thirsty, you're already on your way to trouble. Drink early—before thirst sets in—and often. Experts say that water is perfect for short events, but a commercial sport fluid-replacement drink is preferable for events more than 90 minutes in duration. With either choice, *cold* is best. We want you to play it cool. Drink.

Dance

To Strengthen:	Upper Legs, Hips, and Trunk	1–15
	Lower Legs, Ankles, and Feet	31–35
	If you lift a partner:	
	Shoulders	16–25
	Arms, Elbows, Wrists, and Hands	27–30

Coaches' Notes

We once had a client who asked us if we thought an upcoming dance–exercise class at the local community college would provide a good aerobic program for her. We pointed out that aerobic dance was invented to make cardiovascular workouts fun, and gave her the "thumbs up." When she limped into the clinic less than a week later, she could barely contain her disdain for our stupidity. After all, we had promised her that her heart and lungs would get a good workout, but we had failed to mention that her "body" would have to get involved. (And she wasn't about to ask our opinion on aspirin versus ibuprofen for muscle soreness, even though we sympathetically offered.) Frankly, we were stunned that the client would not make the connection between movement and muscle (or lack thereof), but she's like a lot of us who divide fitness into categories and then tackle them one at a time with no clue that they are interlocked. We restored our credibility with our client by helping her loosen up her body with Active-Isolated Stretching, and when she felt better and could listen to us, we suggested that she start with a strength class and work her way up to aerobic dance when she was strong enough to withstand the rigors of fun.

In recent years, a large percentage of our practice has involved treating injured dancers. Surprised? Don't be. Dancers *are* athletic—strong and flexible. But dancers are sometimes more concerned with form (how they look) than with function (how they get into position), and this lack of understanding puts them at risk. To compound the problem, dancers force their bodies into extreme attitudes that can easily exceed human physical limitations, and they insist on making it all look easy. Injuries are usually the result of creeping, chronic mistakes that gradually sneak up on dancers and knock the legs right out from under them when they can least afford downtime.

The most common injuries in dancers are in the lumbar spine. They result from arching—flexing and extending the back—with improper alignment, and from imbalances in the tendons and muscles. Experts agree that strong abdominals, plus lengthened hip flexors and thoracolumbar fascia, are essential before submitting the spine to the demands of dance without injury. And, of course, proper warm-up is critical in preparing for performance.

Male dancers should be warned about an additional threat of injury: lifting. Not only do men suffer from the "normal" wear and tear that dance places on the body, but many do so while lifting the extra weight of a partner.

Because the disciplines of dance run the gamut from our client's aerobic class at the local community college to professional ballet, tap, and jazz, there is no single formula that can address the physical demands of every facet of the form. But we do know one truth that spans that gamut. Because dancers work out for hours every day and have extraordinary physical capabilities, they can easily assume that they are fit and balanced. Big mistake. Overall fitness requires overall work. And we know of very few dancers who are diligent about total fitness—until they get hurt and end up in our clinic. A few extra minutes of supplementary work to ensure strength, flexibility, and balance go a long way in improving performance capabilities and longevity.

Discus

To Strengthen:	Upper Legs, Hips, and Trunk	1–15
	Shoulders	16–25
	Neck	26
	Arms, Elbows, Wrists, and Hands	27–30
	Lower Legs, Ankles, and Feet	31–35

Coaches' Notes

This used to be the sport of choice for athletes who like to be up on a pedestal. Literally. From its earliest mention in Homeric poetry in 1300 BC until the sport evolved to include a circling technique, discus throwers perched on a narrow column and merely swung the discus back and forth before they released it. In 1910, discus throwers incorporated a one-and-a-half rotation of the body to increase momentum and power, and wisely replaced the pedestal with the 2.5-meter throwing circle on the ground. Even then, athletes knew that the bigger they are, the harder they fall. As effective as the innovations were, frustrated throwers knew that limitations in technique and form were still keeping them from reaching the potential of their power. So, in the 1930s, they increased their standard rotation to a one-and-three-quarters turn and allowed a hop. Although the technique and form we use today have been in place for decades, distances achieved continue to improve through advancements in "human" technologies such as weight training and finely tuned biomechanics.

Strength training is a critical factor in discus throwing, for two reasons: (1) to enable an athlete to hold form in order to balance and harness the considerable forces necessary to sling the discus, and (2) equally important, to prevent injury. It takes muscle to do both.

Medical researchers report that the most common injuries are cuts and bruises to the fingers, followed by sprains and strains of the knee, ankle, shoulder, hip, and back. We won't claim that strength training will "bullet-proof" you so you'll never be injured again, but we can guarantee that it will go a long way toward giving you the structural integrity you need to withstand the rigors of the sport without breaking down. If you think that strength training could help prevent every injury EXCEPT cuts and bruises, think again. Athletes are likely to injure their hands when they grip and release badly because they are not strong enough to control the situation or are off balance and out of position when it's time to release. Strength puts an athlete in control—all the way down to the fingertips.

Mastering discus throwing will not give you a balanced fitness program. Frankly, throwing the discus recruits limited muscle groups into restricted, specific movements each and every time you throw. And, it places stress on one side of your body more than the other. So, if you center your entire fitness program on throwing, you will find yourself physically imbalanced: highly developed in some areas (your right arm, shoulder, and back) and alarmingly weak in others (your left arm, shoulder, back, and both legs). Also, be aware that discus throwing provides little or no cardiovascular conditioning. That's the bad news. The good news is that, if you're like most throwers, you participate in a broad range of related Olympic-style sports, so you no doubt will benefit from other activities. Evaluate your program—*all* the sports you practice—to determine where your deficits are, and round them out with supplemental strength, flexibility, and cardiovascular work.

By the way, the discus throw is the only track-and-field event in which a world's record has never been set in the Olympic Games. Could it be that YOUR time has come?

Fencing

To Strengthen:	Upper Legs, Hips, and Trunk	1–15
	Shoulders	16–25
	Neck	26
	Arms, Elbows, Wrists, and Hands	27–30
	Lower Legs, Ankles, and Feet	31–35

Coaches' Notes

We enjoy it when sports are so infused into our culture that their vocabulary becomes part of our everyday lexicon. Such is the case with fencing. In fencing, "Touché!" means the weapon has made contact with the body. In everyday life, when two people are arguing, "Touché!" means "I scored a point in our argument, but you just got me back. Ouch. Score one for you." More important, "Touché!" is spoken (almost) admiringly by the person who just got verbally gouged and is now acknowledging a superior move by his or her opponent. This simple exchange speaks volumes about sportsmanship and honor that have their roots in fencing.

Fencing began in Europe as sword-fighting in battle and later evolved into the dueling that we know today. In its early days, dueling with sabers was rarely a fight to the death, but merely a contest until one opponent dominated, establishing superiority of skill. A single, nonlethal slash was considered sufficient to win. The winner walked away with his honor in tact. The loser walked away with his spleen unpunctured. Even though a little blood might have been ceremonially shed now and then, fencing was indeed a civilized sport (especially considering the endless possibilities presented by jilted lovers, jealous rages, foggy dawns, and sharp, pointed instruments). And it remains so today, although now no blood is shed.

In spite of the bloodlessness, fencing does present some pretty significant injury risks. We are able to track and study the injuries closely because all sanctioned fencing competitions are required to have on duty medical personnel who file detailed reports on all incidents. Fencing statisticians report that ankle injuries of the trailing leg lead the list. No surprise. There is enormous strain on that leg because it is planted firmly on the floor with the knee bent and the foot turned out. We also see injury of "the total body"—heat-related problems due to exertion, thick uniforms, and (no excuses accepted!) dehydration. "Total body" injury is followed by injuries of the leading leg and foot: strained quadriceps, and trauma to the toes and feet caused by insubstantial shoes and ballistic action. Finally, there is trauma caused by the impact of weapons against the body. The less flexible the weapon, the more serious the bruise. On very rare occasions, there is an accidental puncture.

Training for fencing must be sport-specific. The athlete must be strong, agile, flexible, and balanced in his or her stance. Practice drills develop eye–hand coordination and cardiovascular conditioning. In addition, fencing is one of the few sports that actively promotes a program of mental conditioning to help the athlete maintain focus and emotional control during engagement. The downside to this sport-specific training is that, as a fencer, you tend to be biomechanically imbalanced. One side of your body—the side from which you lead with your weapon—will test much stronger than the other, in both upper and lower extremities. This imbalance renders you vulnerable to injury at all times. A supplemental strength program to balance your body is crucial to maximizing your performance. It will take your weak areas and make them stronger—and take your strong areas and make them awesome. A little extra work and attention to detail will make you a formidable foe on the piste. "En garde!"

Football

To Strengthen:	Upper Legs, Hips, and Trunk	1–15
	Shoulders	16–25
	Neck	26

Coaches' Notes

Thanks to improved playing surfaces, enhanced protective clothing and equipment, and advancing training technologies, football is safer today than it has been at any other time in the history of the sport. Unfortunately, "safe" is a relative term. Football is as safe as any activity where you stand directly in the path of eleven raging men (the size of Mack trucks) on their way to a touchdown. To qualify football as a "collision sport" is to grossly understate the spirit of the sport. It goes beyond collision. In fact, it is the only sport we know that has warning labels on its protective equipment, admonishing the wearer to refrain from using the protective equipment itself to batter another player. (We notice the word "death" on the warning label.) Yet, although we can guarantee injury, every autumn we embrace football as the great American spectator sport. In fact, that's how we recommend that the average person should participate in football: as a spectator.

Having said all this, we know that many people—mostly young men who are not yet aware that they are mortal—will play football every day. If you are one of them, you should be aware of a few things that could spare you a rude encounter with your own mortality. First, work under the leadership of a great coach. Studies have confirmed a direct statistical correlation between an intelligent, experienced head coach with a large staff of assistants, and a reduced risk of team injuries. Second, wear every bit of protective clothing and equipment you can find. And finally, come to the playing field in good condition and rested. Statistics indicate that the fewest injuries take place in the first quarter. It's no coincidence. Players are fresh and better able to meet the demands of the game than they will be later. Also, if you're a Sunday afternoon player, save the beer drinking for the postgame barbecue. An out-of-control player—too out-of-shape, too fatigued, and too impaired to play—is a danger to himself and everyone on the gridiron.

Listing injuries related to playing football would be an exercise in futility. You name it, it's on the list. (Medical units carry *bolt cutters* in their field kits. Tell you anything?) And statistically, it makes no difference whether you are playing offense or defense. They present equal opportunity risks. Pressed to name the number one bonecrusher? The tackle. No surprise.

Listing physical requirements and training strategies for playing is also difficult because each position has its own specific challenges. Strength training is critically important for any football player. It takes power to handle the game. But being strong is only one component of a good fitness program. It is also important that you build and maintain cardiovascular fitness for endurance to be able to sustain energy throughout the game and, equally important, run. Cardiovascular work offers a sort of "Catch-22" in the thinking of a football player, where physical size counts. If you participate in aggressive cardiovascular workouts, your fat stores will drop and you'll lose bulk. You'll be stronger, faster, healthier, and more energetic. But if you get smaller, you'll get pounded by the bigger guys. On the other hand, if you don't do the cardiovascular work, you'll be able to store body fat and be physically larger, but you'll be slow on the field and will have less stamina. Also, there are long-term health concerns, such as cardiovascular diseases, associated with carrying too much body fat. See the catch? It's up to you and your trainers to find the balance that gives you the best of each end of the catch.

Football is a game of strategy, cunning, courage, camaraderie, and stunning athletic prowess. As thrilling as it is, however, it is also one of the most dangerous sports we play. Caution is advised. We asked one trainer to tell us what he thought the number one football injury was. He replied, "Football injury. Isn't that redundant?"

Golf

Coaches' Notes

Years ago, we sat on an airplane with an engineer from MIT who was working on quantifying the "perfect" golf swing. When we asked why the simple golf swing should command the attention of such a prestigious university, the engineer said that the golf swing is anything but simple. It is, in fact, an engineering marvel—one of those biomechanical conundrums that intrigue scientists who can't explain it and frustrate duffers who can't master it. He said that a "perfect" golf swing appeared to be such a complex function that it actually should be physically impossible. To swing and hit the ball to the green time after time should require a calibrated pendulum surgically mounted between the throat and the chest. He remarked that it's amazing that an utterly human golfer (with no pendulum) can gauge distance, topography, and weather conditions, set her sites on a far-off hole, wind up her entire body, raise a slender club overhead, then uncoil while sweeping the club down to strike a tiny ball, send it flying to a tiny target beyond sight, and succeed in getting it there. But scientists like this engineer and those of us who work in sports know a secret. The human being is a miraculous creature, capable of galvanizing body and spirit to accomplish impossible things all the time. Besides, until that night on the plane, no one bothered to tell us that "perfect" golf swings are impossible.

Sports medicine experts who have studied the golf swing and measured the forces that the body uses in all phases of the game point out that golf does not rely on strength as much as it does on highly refined motor skills and flexibility. While there appears to be little or no correlation between muscular strength and the ability to hit the ball farther or longer, experts report that the stronger a player is, the more consistently he is able to strike the ball and the longer he will be able to maintain that consistency. Also, muscular weakness makes a player prone to injury. Particularly vulnerable are the knees and lower back, which take the stress of rotation when a golfer winds up and then uncoils during a swing.

As much fun as golf is, frankly it's not great exercise. To be really fit, you will have to supplement your game with strength training (concentrate on those shoulders!), stretching, and cardiovascular work. There are some ways, however, to use the sport to help. If you are able, leave the golf cart in the garage and walk. Carry or pull your own clubs. Use "down" time between shots to stretch and keep moving. (But avoid annoying your partners and disrupting their concentration. Nothing is more irritating than trying to make a difficult shot with a guy doing jumping jacks and grunting behind you. In fact, we're pretty sure this is grounds for justifiable homicide in some states.)

For a sport as gentle as golf, injuries are surprisingly common. The problem is not that the sport is so strenuous, but that many golfers underestimate the risks and approach the sport out of shape. Most injuries are due to overuse, improper biomechanics, and sloppy technique. Fortunately, all of these are avoidable with moderation, physical training, proper equipment, and good coaching. Golfers have even more motivation to stay healthy. In spite of tried and true rehabilitation methods specific to golfing injuries, half of those golfers injured are bothered by the injury for a long time. Recovery tends to be frustratingly slow.

We would be remiss in the discussion of golf injuries if we did not mention emotional distress. No, we're not talking about falling into a funk over a missed shot. In this case, we're talking about physical injury caused by a player in a blind rage or, conversely, in the throes of ecstasy. An alarming number of injuries (and even deaths) occur when a player rampages out of control. The anecdotes about absurd incidents—both accidental and deliberate—are endless. A player celebrates a great shot by throwing her club into the air; it aims its descent at the bald spot of the nearest golfer. A player hurls his golf bag against a tree in a fit of temper and forgets to let go before the moment of impact. It shatters his wrists, and then, as the bag rebounds off the tree, it slams him in the face, knocking him to the ground and breaking his nose. A player has missed one too many shots and is sick of hearing suggestions; he bounces a ball off the forehead of his caddie. And so on and so forth. You get the picture. Remember, golf is supposed to be fun and relaxing. You're out in the fresh air and sunshine, playing with your friends. So keep it light.

Gymnastics

Coaches' Notes

For our client Jean Ketchum, one of the great delights of the Olympic Games is women's gymnastics, where elfin, pony-tailed women prance into the arena and take command of center stage. Jean once remarked that they're like molecules of plutonium: each tiny, jam-packed powerhouse has within her such explosive energy that she can cause a meltdown. And Jean's right. That's what a great gymnast does. Jean Ketchum came to us after the 1996 Olympic Games because she wanted to be a gymnast. The problem was that she was a 43-year-old woman who had yet to master a somersault.

We've never been trainers who dash the dreams of an aspiring athlete, so we told Jean that we could help her train as a gymnast, but we would encourage more modest goals than making the next American Olympic team. It's nothing personal. In fact, gymnastics is one of the few sports where the athletes begin at a very early age—childhood—and peak when the rest of us are just warming up. Emerging technologies and training techniques might advance our perceptions of human performance potential, and we might see older athletes in the future, but for right now, gymnastics at the Olympic level is the exclusive domain of the very young. This doesn't mean that there's not room for the rest of us outside the Olympic venues and professional arenas. Indeed, gymnastics can be a lot of fun and great exercise. (Jean, by the way, is doing very well.)

Because the disciplines of the sport are so diverse, general suggestions and remarks are difficult. But all aspects of gymnastics—both men's and women's—do have one thing in common: they place huge demands on the body that require total mental and physical control. For this reason, training is critical. And so, therefore, is the coach. As the maneuvers increase in degrees of difficulty, so does the skill required to teach them properly (and safely!), so we encourage you to work with the best coach you can find and to be willing to move to a more advanced coach when your skill level matches or exceeds the capabilities of your current coach. (If you catch him or her thumbing frantically through the book while you're upside down in midair, it's time to pack your chalk and find another training facility.)

Studies all concur that the most dangerous gymnastic event (for both men and women) is floor exercise. Sprained ankles and strained knees lead women's injuries statistics; and sprained and strained ankles, knees, shoulders, and wrists lead men's. Most injuries take place in practice and most occur in incidents where there were no spotters. Finally, it appears that the more elite the athlete, the more difficult the maneuver, and the more likely an injury. The solution is to practice your craft as safely as possible. Be certain that you are physically trained to perform the maneuvers, sufficiently warmed up, and rested, and have a spotter standing by.

To be truly fit, you have to have cardiovascular fitness for endurance, and be healthy, well, strong, and flexible. In gymnastics, the drive for flexibility is a double-edged sword as the athlete pushes to reach the end ranges of motion. It is critically important that you have muscular strength to support your movements. Pushing your body to flex and extend into an impressive position is one thing. Having the power to get yourself right to the "edge" (no farther!) and (more important!) back is quite another. The more flexible you are in gymnastics, the stronger you have to be.

Adding to the problem of insufficient muscular strength is insufficient skeletal integrity, particularly in very young people. The skeleton is a dynamic, living organism, constantly building to match a growing body, then rebuilding itself throughout a lifetime, in direct response to structural stresses (or "load"). When a growth spurt temporarily renders the skeleton a little vulnerable and a gymnast hammers it in a workout, the bone may not be able to withstand the pounding or to rebuild fast enough to fortify itself. The consequence is an unstable structure, the symptoms of which are frequently manifested in the spine. Low back pain, disk injuries and failures, and fractures of the spine signal that the skeleton is not mature enough to support the maneuvers. The difficulty is compounded by weak abdominals (common, even in gymnasts!), which force the spine to take more of the load in flexion and extension than is necessary. The gymnast needs to slow down and ease up.

Caution: A special word to women gymnasts: Nature deposits a layer of fat around the muscles of all women. You're trying to be as light as possible, but dieting to drop your percentage of body fat below 16 percent may delay menses; or, if you're already menstruating, it may cause your estrogen levels to diminish, possibly resulting in your losing estrogen's cardioprotective properties, developing amenorrhea, and running an increased risk of osteoporosis. Every woman is different, so you and your physician will want to monitor your body carefully and make intelligent decisions that take into consideration the long-term consequences of dieting.

Hammer Throw

Coaches' Notes

Hammer throwing has its roots in Irish antiquity, but it is a sport that continues to evolve as technology and our understanding of physics suggest greater potential for performance. As late as the 1960s, innovations were still being introduced and accepted into international competitions, the latest being four turns within the seven-foot circle.

To us, hammer throwing is an interesting sport because its physics are "backward" at first glance. Instead of propelling the object you're throwing, you actually lead the hammer as it circles and gains the momentum it needs to achieve distance when it's released. But, while you're leading the whirling hammer, you're also the power behind the throw. Not only must you be strong, coordinated, and flexible, but you must also possess a superior understanding of physics. You actually transfer force from your legs, through your hips, up your back, through your shoulders, and down your arms to the chain AHEAD of the hammer. Each successive circle is a little faster and moves the hammer higher. With flexed knees, you lean back against the centrifugal forces generated by the weight, mass, and velocity of the hammer as it whirls. And, at a precise moment of decision that can only be described as metaphysically inspired, you release the hammer and wait for applause. It is really quite a phenomenon: simple and elegant at the same time.

Hammer throwing places enormous physical demands on the thrower. Strength training is generalized and intense, for no part of the body is less critical than any other. We would remind you, however, that training for hammer throwing does not provide a superior cardiovascular workout, and you will want to supplement your program with an activity like running, swimming, or cycling.

Sports medicine experts classify injuries related to the sport into two categories: (1) those caused by physical mistakes and (2) those caused by equipment failure. Fortunately, you have a lot of control over both. Proper conditioning and warm-up will help you protect particularly vulnerable areas—shoulders, back, hips, abdominals, and neck—from injuries attributable to exertion, overuse, and trauma. In addition, you will want to protect your wire from any kinking, crimping, or wear that may compromise its structural integrity. Check it before every throw. Nothing is more dangerous in this sport than having the wire break while an athlete is circling with the hammer in extension. At the moment of release, it will throw the athlete backward. Also, to protect yourself before you begin the circle, clear the ground of debris and even out any irregularities in the surface. And finally, make certain that there is no one around you whom you can bean when you release. Many athletes make sure that the area in front of them is clear, but we like to consider the possibility that a faulty release could propel the hammer in a direction that they least expect. We coach our athletes to visually sweep a full arc around the throwing circle and make sure that, no matter where that Buick is parked, it's out of the line of fire.

Handball

To Strengthen:	Upper Legs, Hips, and Trunk	1–15
	Shoulders	16–25
	Neck	26
	Arms, Elbows, Wrists, and Hands	27–30
	Lower Legs, Ankles, and Feet	31–35

Coaches' Notes

"Street sports" have a special place in our hearts. (Hey. We're New Yorkers. Go figure.) And handball is one of the best. In its essence, it's truly "mano a mano": two ferocious competitors, a wall, and a rocket-paced ball. Add padded gloves and shatterproof eyewear for protection, and you have the perfect game.

If simplicity is handball's beauty, it is also its downside. Ironically, the absence of equipment—specifically, a paddle or racquet—allows the specter of injury to arise more frequently than we would like to see. Let us explain. When we put a paddle or a racquet in the hand of an athlete, it slows the shoulder–arm action down with its weight and resistance. But in handball, without these "brakes," the athlete engages in a sort of full-acceleration "snap" or "slap" at the ball, violently engaging muscles from the back through the shoulder down the arm through the wrist to the hand. For a maneuver so large, the movement is quick and overt. There needs to be a perfect strike, so the player adds a split-second torque in the arc to position and brace the palm of his hand to make contact. Yet, when his hand connects with the ball, the impact needed to return the ball is so light that the follow-through on this movement is barely slowed down. It can be a jarring, wrenching moment for a hard hitter. Strength and flexibility training can make a big difference in tempering the power and coordinating the stroke.

In addition to shoulder, elbow, and wrist injuries caused by the action necessary to connect with the ball, the simplicity of the sport has one more insidious consequence. It deceives players into thinking that the sport is easy. Simple does not mean easy. Although the rules are easy, the sport is killer. Make sure you're in condition to play before you step out onto the court and challenge your competitor. And remember to warm up properly.

One of our nonnegotiable rules for handball is that you have to wear the proper shoes. Forget running shoes. They might be really comfortable and look ferocious, but they are engineered for moving an athlete forward. They are not forgiving when you try to move side to side and backward, or (heaven forbid!) pivot. If you initiate any move other than forward, the waffling pattern sculpted on the sole will grab the surface, just as the manufacturer designed it to do. You will end up on your face (and totally humiliated because it will happen when there's no one to blame it on). Try specially designed racquet sport shoes, basketball shoes, or aerobic shoes. No matter which you choose, look for good support, comfort, and, equally important, permission from the shoes to move in any direction. One of the real dangers in handball is "shin splints"—an overuse injury to the shins from micro-tearing of the muscles and tendons that run along the bone at the front of the leg (tibia). Shin splints are caused by pounding, and their origins are often in feet that are weak and inflexible and in shoes that are cruel and unusual. They are painful reminders that an athlete has work to do.

We insist that you wear protective eyewear. Handball is amazingly fast-paced and, although we want you to keep your eye on the ball, we don't mean it literally. Damage to the eye is cited by sports medicine experts as the most dangerous injury in the sport.

High Jump

To Strengthen:	Upper Legs, Hips, and Trunk	1–15
	Shoulders	16–25
	Lower Legs, Ankles, and Feet	31–35

Coaches' Notes

No competitive athlete likes to flop. Except one: the high jumper. This sport, although one of the ancient sports of the Olympiad, continues to evolve and incorporate innovations in equipment and technique. And this evolution brings us to the Fosbury Flop, a backward soar and dive over the bar introduced by American Dick Fosbury in the 1968 Olympic Games in Mexico City. At the time, it was more revolutionary than evolutionary and it set the sport on its ear—well, on its back, anyway.

Jumpers, impressed by the increased height afforded by this unusual torque, embraced the technique. It quickly became the competitive standard. But during its first years, the Fosbury Flop caused problems for jumpers who were ecstatic with the jump but less than pleased with the landing. For one thing, the jumper was backward when he or she cleared the bar. There was no visual contact with the mat. So the moment of impact was liable to be a bit of a shock—a split second before or after the jumper expected to hit. And worse, the jumper was landing on the back of the head, on a mat that frankly was not designed to cushion such a hit. Spinal injuries and head injuries sometimes resulted from bad landings. It was a tricky irony. We had the most effective technique for attaining height and nailing a clean jump, but it was a back-breaker. Necessity is the mother of invention, as they say. Rather than abandon the Flop, the sport merely advanced the technology used to design the mats for better shock absorption. Additionally, we learned to apply the basic physics of impact and further developed our ability to diffuse energy when an athlete lands. Today, jumpers are trained to mitigate the force of impact by throwing both arms back to strike the mat a split second before their head and back make contact.

Although injuries to the back and head are the most common, the Fosbury Flop can sometimes deliver a second source of injury to high jumpers. The jumper runs straight to the bar, but in order to pivot around to fly backward, he or she must transfer that forward momentum of the run to vertical lift. It's done by veering off the straightforward run and using the last steps of the approach to angle the body so that the back is to the bar. It's a sort of "J" pattern: a straight run followed by an arc. The forces are enormous on the legs and feet. The result of a misstep combined with weak or inflexible anatomy is a high incidence of sprained ankles.

Sports medicine experts recommend that you make every effort to train for each aspect of the sport with individual attention to detail. Further, they advise that you should never come to the field unless you're warmed up and rested. And finally, they suggest that you become proficient in all jumping techniques and alternate them in practice, saving the most dangerous for the highest bars.

We would like to add that training for the high jump is not the perfect fitness program. Training for this one event will leave you with some serious imbalances and deficits. Fortunately, the high jump is almost always part of a more comprehensive track-and-field menu, and the inclusion of other disciplines will help you develop a more well-rounded fitness program. You should plan to add supplemental training in strength (take a look at upper body), aerobics (sprinting a few yards will not deliver a good cardiovascular program), and flexibility (research has conclusively demonstrated that the injury rate in high jump is due in part to inflexibility of hips, ankles, and spine). Now, go flop.

Hiking

Coaches' Notes

A friend of ours recently observed, "Walking is basic transportation, but hiking is a commitment." We aren't sure that his declaration clearly defines the differences between the two, but it certainly does nudge the distinctions. Hiking is walking for entertainment, education, and exercise. It's done outside in wide open spaces (for example, up and down a mountain rather than up and down the hall), and it frequently involves special footwear and equipment.

We like hiking because it's a good strength workout for hips, back, legs, and feet. Additionally, it can be a good aerobic workout if you turn up the intensity of your hike. In fact, it's this ability to moderate intensity that makes hiking such a valuable workout component. At sea level, on flat ground, at strolling pace, and carrying nothing, hiking can be an easy workout. At altitude, up a 90-degree graded trail, at a scorching pace, and carrying a 35-pound pack, hiking can be a killer workout. The choice is entirely up to you. One sport, variable levels.

Although hiking can be a good workout, it's not a complete one. Upper back, shoulders, and arms are rarely engaged to their full capacity. You'll want to supplement your hiking program with strength work. Also, you're rarely in position to be able to hike on a daily basis. If you're like most of us, the sport is reserved for weekends at most and vacations at least. We don't have to remind you that infrequent workouts yield inconsistent (nearly accidental) gains in fitness. Engaging in regular exercise that stresses muscle development, flexibility, and cardiovascular work will give you the fitness you need to enjoy the hiking (and the confidence to outdistance a bear).

Little is more important in hiking than the selection of your footwear. You should invest in shoes or boots that are manufactured for hiking. These are comfortable, designed to support your feet on uneven surfaces over long distances, and able to help keep your feet dry by creating a miraculous high-tech moisture barrier that keeps outside dampness from seeping in, yet allows sweat to wick out. A dry foot is less likely to develop "hot-spots" or blisters. You'll want to wear sports socks designed to assist wicking. Some people who are particularly blister-prone choose to wear two pairs of socks at the same time. The theory is that the two socks—one against the foot and one against the boot—slide against each other and absorb the surface friction between the foot and the boot. Other blister-prone hikers put a thin barrier of petroleum jelly on the soles of their feet and toes before putting on socks. Be sure to wear ALL the socks you're going to hike in when you try on new boots or shoes. If your boots don't fit well, your toes will jam against the end of the toe box on the downhill. Equally annoying, your heels will jam against the back of the boot on the uphill. And, even worse, your gait will be unsteady as you struggle within your boot to find firm footing with each step. An ill-fitting boot can cause you great discomfort—and injury.

If you're going to be out more than an hour, you'll want to carry supplies. For short trips, you'll need the basics: water, a little first-aid kit, a compass, and a whistle. (Phil refuses to leave the base camp without his cell phone.) For longer trips, you'll need to add the survival stuff, including food, shelter, clothing, and supplies. Most of the time, a hiker will carry extras in a pack: little rucksacks for light loads and hip-cinched backpacks with shoulder suspension systems for heavy ones. Carrying anything, no matter how small, does two things to your workout: it adds weight that increases your load (good thing!) and it adds that weight in places that unbalance your natural gait (bad thing!). When you put the pack on your back, it tends to pull you over backward. The heavier the pack, the more insistent the pull. To compensate for the addition—even while standing still—you'll automatically lean forward at the waist and tighten your lower abdominals. Muscles in your lower back contract to keep you upright, causing your pelvis to rock slightly forward to arch your back and take the pressure off. Any oblique movement, such as raising one leg to move forward or reaching down to pick something up, will cause an instantaneous chain reaction of compensatory muscle contractions and adjustments as your body struggles to maintain equilibrium. The compensations might be so slight that you will not even notice them, but your body will fatigue more quickly than you expect and, at the end of the day, you might have aches and pains, the sources of which you can't quite pinpoint. And, of course, it goes without saying that when you tamper with your center of gravity, you're less stable than you think you are. With a pack on, it won't take much more to knock you off balance. Be careful. The answer is to be strong enough to support the weight of your pack. If you're going to go on a long hike with a heavy pack, you might train by taking shorter hikes with increasing amounts of weight in the pack. One of our friends carries bricks in his pack (adding one more every day) for the first few weeks of his program and then graduates to cinder blocks before he makes his yearly trek into bear country. By the time he hits the mountain, he's in great shape. He developed this system after his first trip—a self-described two-week brutal march straight into hell. He found himself sitting on a rock on the second morning, pawing through his pack and asking himself the all-important questions: "Do I *really* need this heavy food? How necessary is this water? And this sleeping bag . . . hey, do I *really* need it?" Today, he not only carries all the same stuff he had on the first trip, but he's added one more thing. Training.

Horseback Riding

To Strengthen:	Upper Legs, Hips, and Trunk	1–15
	Shoulders	16–25
	Neck	26
	Arms, Elbows, Wrists, and Hands	27–30

Coaches' Notes

In all the world of sports, horseback riding is unique in that your success as an athlete directly depends on the performance of a partner who weighs ten times more than you do, but has only one-tenth of your intelligence. (Easy, you pairs skaters . . . .) Contrasts notwithstanding, riders and horses have been "matches made in heaven" for more than five thousand years of recorded history. Today, as it has always been, horseback riding is as much a love affair as it is a sport. In this relationship, you might perform as a single unit, but there are two athletes to consider in all aspects of your work together.

Safety is the prime directive. We find it chilling that, unlike most other sports, the research published on horseback riding injuries is focused not on biomechanical mistakes, but on trauma caused by accidents. This *is* a dangerous sport for both rider and horse. The very act of riding is to perch a rider in the saddle. It's a balancing act that changes second by second. Stability is a fragile illusion, because gripping the saddle with your knees, pressuring the stirrups with your feet, and settling into your center of gravity do NOT cement you into position. One stumble and you're on the ground. The great irony is that, when you mount your horse, your most vulnerable point (that one on top of your head) is the farthest from the ground and gains the most momentum on its way down. For this reason, we insist that you wear protective headgear at all times. A ten-gallon hat might look sexy, but its shock-absorbing capabilities are more shocking than absorbing. A helmet will help protect you from head trauma. And speaking of equipment, safety is directly linked to tack that's in good condition. Tack suffers a lot of wear and tear, so you'll want to inspect yours every time you use it. Regular maintenance and replacement of worn gear should be high priorities. By the way, equestrian statisticians point out that one can be injured in a horseback riding accident without even being on the horse.

For example, the horse can step on a person or mash him against the fence or bite him on the arm, or—frankly, the list is as endless as the possibilities presented by a one-ton horse dancing around a careless buckaroo.

Horseback riders tend to be in good shape not because riding is such a good workout, but because taking care of horses is hard work and keeps a person active on a daily basis. But not everyone is fortunate enough to get to work that hard. If you're boarding your horse and letting someone else have all the fun, you'll need to consider supplemental fitness work. Although most riders tend to be strong in their legs and hips, they are notoriously underdeveloped in the upper body, shoulders, and arms. (News flash. Holding the reins just doesn't give you a good workout.) And you'll need a good flexibility program. Under many circumstances during the ride, your body (particularly your hips and spine) takes a pounding. A flexible rider literally becomes a spring—able to absorb and spring back from the jarring. Also, being flexible means that you have greater ranges of motion and can change your position more quickly and more completely. All this comes in handy when you need to make a quick escape or engineer a rapid dismount without thinking. And finally, in order to be really fit, you must supplement your riding with cardiovascular work. (Unless you're running alongside your horse, you're getting no aerobic work at the stable.)

Hurdles

To Strengthen:	Upper Legs, Hips, and Trunk	1–15
	Shoulders	16–25
	Neck	26
	Lower Legs, Ankles, and Feet	31–35

Coaches' Notes

When we hear the expression "clearing hurdles" used in daily life, we all understand that it means "overcoming problems thrown in the path." When the difficulty of a sport is so universally understood that it becomes a metaphor for triumph over adversity, that's a sport that truly deserves our respect. Hurdles is that sport.

We particularly enjoy hurdles because it is a practice in the art of deception. To the casual observer, it looks like a jumping event. But we're going to let you in on a secret. It's not jumping at all. It's a sprinting event with one exaggerated airborne step thrown in. As it does for all sprinters, the heat begins when you fire off your starting block, and accelerate down your lane. The mechanics, at this point, are identical to the sprint. Suddenly, a hurdle looms in your path. You transfer your sprint gait into flight by using your back leg to push off and extending your leading leg over the hurdle. You press forward by keeping your arms in front of you and leaning in the direction you're running. It's a tricky set of maneuvers. If you lean too far forward or too quickly, you'll nail the hurdle. If you lean too far backward or too slowly, you'll knock your center of gravity toward the back leg and fall. If you get it right, your trailing leg flexes (the knee bends) to clear the top of the hurdle. Nearly simultaneously, you direct your front leg toward the ground until your foot makes contact with the track and you launch back into the standard sprint—to make up for the acceleration lost in flight, and to work up the power you'll need to blaze down the lane and get over the next hurdle. Just when you thought things couldn't get any more difficult, remember that you have to be proficient in clearing the hurdle using *either leg* as the lead. (We think this is like telling a right-handed person that she has great penmanship, but she won't be able to write another word until she can do it just as beautifully with her left hand as well.) Now you see why clearing the hurdle has become a metaphor for overcoming problems—big problems.

Flexibility is a critical factor in success. Being able to snap from a full-out sprint into an extension of the front leg and a flexion of the back leg in the blink of an eye requires command of a full range of motion. The consequences of failure are two: either you will strain or tear something, or you'll be on your face on the track with a medic hovering over you and shouting, "Get the Jaws of Life! We have a hurdle to remove!" The duration of a hurdles heat is relatively short, but the effort is intense. No question that you'll become exhausted. (If you don't, you're not giving the event your best effort.) Research confirms that fatigue works insidiously to shorten your stride so that you run more slowly and must work even harder to compensate to gain lift, extension, and flexion. Flexibility will help offset this inevitable deterioration. Sports medicine files are bulging with case studies of injuries endemic to hurdlers, and most of them are related to inflexibility. You can avoid this with a good program. (May we recommend Active-Isolated Stretching?)

The other area of injury is trauma—injury due to accident. The more skilled you are, the less frequently you will crash. But frankly, we know of no one who has not clipped a hurdle and taken a bad tumble—or maybe a thousand tumbles. It goes with the territory. Perfect shoes designed to absorb shock (particularly in the heel), perfect surfaces (even, soft, and clear of debris), perfect equipment (regulation hurdles set up in the right direction), and perfect training (including sprinting, strength training, and flexibility) will minimize accidents.

Ice Hockey

To Strengthen:	Upper Legs, Hips, and Trunk	1–15
	Shoulders	16–25
	Neck	26
	Arms, Elbows, Wrists, and Hands	27–30
	Lower Legs, Ankles, and Feet	31–35

Coaches' Notes

Historians theorize that hockey originated in ancient Europe as a diversion for bored shepherds who strapped broken animal bones onto the bottom of their feet and took to the ice. Although the sport has evolved since those early days, one thing remains constant: broken bones. Today, hockey players skate on metal blades and save the breaking for their own bones after they get onto the ice. Unlike athletes in other contact sports, who are more likely to get hurt during practice, hockey players are more than three times as likely to get hurt during actual games, and of those players injured, more than three-fourths of them will get hurt as a result of contact. At first glance, it doesn't make sense. But, this is hockey. The very nature of this game is aggression. Add skaters who sear across the ice at speeds in excess of 30 mph, a puck that rockets at 100 mph with impact force up to 1,200 pounds, hard ice, confined space, and sticks, and you have all the ingredients for a sure-fire bone-cruncher—and an exciting game.

Injury rates notwithstanding, hockey skating is distinct from all other skating in its unique combination of the athletic skills required. Hockey skaters have to be able to power skate in all directions, change directions second-by-second, and stop on a dime. In fact, so famous is this ability to stop that snow skiing has adapted a similar technique and calls it the "hockey stop." A skier comes flying down the mountain without making any attempt to brake. Within a few feet of the target, the skier suddenly lifts the back of the skis, pivots, digs them in, and sprays snow as the run comes to an abrupt and dramatic conclusion (just in time to administer CPR to the person showered with snow and scared to death).

Hockey—the sport itself and how the players use their bodies—has been studied extensively. Of particular interest are the unique demands placed on the hips and legs of hockey players. Hockey has moves and forces that are not found in other sports—for example, snapping the hip into flexion while extending the knee, generating force ratios that are the greatest found in sports. Supplemental strength work pays huge dividends in athletic performance and injury prevention.

Equally important is cardiovascular fitness. Largely considered to be endurance athletes, hockey players—with stopping and starting during play—have neither the cardiovascular benefit of an aerobic workout nor the high-intensity benefits of an anaerobic one. It's ironic, because scientists have demonstrated a direct correlation between cardiovascular fitness (a high maximum VO_2 level) and performance. We would like to add that the ability to carry and use oxygen forestalls fatigue and hastens recovery after a tough game. In other words, if you supplement your workout program with specific cardiovascular training, you'll do better on the ice. Guaranteed.

Hockey is seriously demanding, but does not deliver a great workout. Sports medicine experts warn against thinking that time on the ice is getting you into shape. In between seasons and in between games, you have to be diligent in strength, flexibility, and cardiovascular work. Not only will you play better, but you will tip the odds of injury in the other direction.

A final note: Never underestimate the dangers—as well as the joys—inherent in playing hockey. Wear every bit of protective equipment you can find. Play to win but, more important, play safely and intelligently.

Jumping: Long Jump and Triple Jump

To Strengthen:	Upper Legs, Hips, and Trunk	1–15
	Shoulders	16–25
	Neck	26
	Lower Legs, Ankles, and Feet	31–35

Coaches' Notes

A couple of weeks ago, one of our track-and-field clients remarked that his apartment was "just a hop, skip and a jump" from the track. We laughed because not only had he used a familiar colloquialism to describe a short distance, but he had also, unintentionally, perfectly described his event, the triple jump. (By the way, it takes a lot longer to get to the triple jump than it does to get from our friend's apartment to the track. The "triple" is a complex and elegant sport.)

Essentially, triple jump is, as we said, "a hop, skip, and a jump." You make three progressive moves forward, each higher and longer than the one before. This sequential amplification is made possible by using your arms to drive your body up, and using your lower body as a sort of spring: coiling and recoiling, storing and then releasing energy forward and upward at each moment of impact. The final arc—the "jump"—concludes the event as you land on both feet. Your knees bend to absorb the shock, and forward momentum drives you to your knees. You thrust your hands straight out and to the ground to stop the forward roll. (Hopefully, at this point, you rise from the sand to thunderous applause and a new record.)

Most injuries take place on the landings. Feet, ankles, and knees are particularly vulnerable—for two reasons. First, any physical imbalance or off-kilter flight will result in an uneven landing for which the body will attempt a series of rather unattractive but valiant compensations. The result can be a strain, sprain, or fracture. And second, no matter how perfect the landings are, repeated impact sometimes results in irritations and overuse injuries such as tendinitis. But the landings are not the only dangerous moments. Injuries in triple jump also involve lower back and glute pain caused by lifting off the ground on one foot and snapping the torso and hips around into a forward lean. Driving the arms up to facilitate lift can cause strain in the chest, shoulders, and upper back. Other common complaints are shin splints and pain at the back of the knee (caused by increased stride length and inflexible feet and ankles that cannot absorb the shock).

Related to the triple jump is the long jump, also called the running broad jump. It is a sentimental favorite of ours because it is one of the five original Olympic events. The long jump gets its name from the airborne phase of the jump. Because the approach is a full-out sprint, the momentum after liftoff tends to carry the jumper for an impressive distance. In fact, some jumpers continue to run in midair rather than disrupt that pattern. Other jumpers tuck their knees in an effort to keep their feet off the ground until the last possible nanosecond. No matter how you fly, the landing has to be perfect: feet first, knees slightly bent to absorb shock, and center of gravity passing over your feet until you are firmly on the ground. As in the triple jump, many jumpers brake that forward momentum on the landing by thrusting their arms out and planting their hands in the sand. As important as braking at the end is, it's also important to learn NOT to brake at the beginning. One of the truly valuable lessons in injury prevention is to learn to recognize an approach that is going to fail, make a decision to pull out, and (here's the hard part) defy all logic as you continue to run over the springboard and right into the pit. Anything short of this will put you at serious risk of ankle and knee injury.

Because these events are short in duration, you can't count on them to provide your workout. Fortunately, if you're like most track-and-field athletes, you practice the jumps in concert with other events that will afford you more opportunity for training. No matter. You will want to supplement your training with cardiovascular work (running!), strength training for full control, and flexibility to give you full ranges of motion and maximum shock absorption in impact. No excuses. The fitness center is probably just a "hop, skip, and a jump" from the track, right?

Kayaking

To Strengthen:	Upper Legs, Hips, and Trunk	1–15
	Shoulders	16–25
	Arms, Elbows, Wrists, and Hands	27–30
	Lower Legs, Ankles, and Feet	31–35

Coaches' Notes

To quote a Native American proverb: "Every day you spend on the water is another day you add to your life." In the case of kayaking, we would like to modify it to read: "Every day you spend on, in, over, under, upside down, inside out, and up your nose in water is another day you add to your life and subtract from the life of a Wharton." As heart-stopping as kayaking can be, it's also a spectacular sport that builds great athletes.

Mastering the kayak starts when you discover that your boat is a limber, facile, responsive extension of your body. We recommend that you begin your training by becoming adept at basic techniques in still water and advancing to moving water BEFORE you tackle whitewater or surf. A methodical, intelligent approach is a safe one. Like all paddling sports, kayaking is fun on a great variety of levels, from beginner to advanced. Literally, it's "different strokes for different folks." Kayaking can be an easy, relaxing activity where rhythmic paddling and sight-seeing are the orders of the day. Or it can be a rocketing roller coaster ride that strains your body to its limits and kicks your adrenaline up into overdrive. Without question, kayaking is a versatile fitness tool— and great fun.

When you paddle, your pulling arm is retroverted from a lateral position and lowered, with your elbow and wrist flexed upward. In opposition, your pushing arm is gradually extended by the back of your upper arm and raised by the muscles in the back of your shoulder. The entire pull is supported by muscles low in your back and hips—your trunk rotators. Your legs extend in front of you, from your hips, to stabilize and equalize the forces generated by your upper body as you paddle and torque.

Most injuries in kayaking fall into two categories: trauma and overuse injuries. We'll first dispatch the "trauma" issue by saying this: don't run into things, don't let things run into you, and don't hit bottom.

Now, moving on to overuse injuries, there are two major areas of difficulty in kayaking: paddling and sitting. How, you ask, can sitting causing an injury? Very simply. Few other sports are as demanding on the upper body as kayaking and NONE of them makes those demands from a seated position in a cockpit. Frankly, human beings weren't designed to handle that kind of load from a seat. Because a kayaker is locked into the fanny-down/back-up/legs-out position, the lower back really takes a beating. Not only does it serve as a sort of pivot point and command center for the coordination of incredible forces above it, but it also anchors the entire body below. Injured kayakers present with back irritations, strains, sprains, disk herniation, and sciatic nerve compression—all injuries of overuse. In addition to back injuries, we see nerve impingement in shoulders and forearms. This happens when the repetitive motion of paddling causes muscles to swell and compress nerves, resulting in pain and numbness. Also, we see irritated tendons, strains, and sprains in shoulders, arms, and wrists. And, because of the repetitive motion of paddling and the unrelenting pressure of the paddles on the hands, kayakers experience the same sequence of debilitating symptoms that characterizes carpal tunnel syndrome: fatigue first, then irritation followed by pain, and finally numbness and loss of motor control. As if all this were not bad enough, acrobatic kayakers who cartwheel in rodeo and surfing have spawned a whole new generation of injuries. Sports medicine physicians are now seeing muscle tears in the lower back, intercostal muscles, and elbow joints. Most injuries can be avoided (or minimized) by laying in the basic skills before you advance to the next level of difficulty, proper physical training, and adequate warm-up before you snap in.

As wonderful as kayaking is, it is not a complete fitness program. The physical demands are enormous, and you'll really enhance your performance if you supplement your kayaking with flexibility and strength work. Kayakers are known for strong upper bodies accompanied by weak hips and legs. It makes sense that the hips and legs would fall behind the upper body in development because of the limited range of motion imposed by the cockpit and the lack of function during the sport. If you're to be a well-rounded athlete, you're going to have to work hard on dry land. Also, there's a lot to be said for the benefits of endurance and stamina that follow a good cardiovascular program. (You want to be able to hold your breath a long time after the kayak flies, don't you?!?) We recommend that you add running, cycling, or swimming to your workout regimen. (Maybe swimming would be the best for you. You never know when you'll need to be good at it!) Finally, we want to caution you (as we do all athletes who engage in sports that tend to be seasonal) to take care of yourself and maintain a good fitness base in the off-season. When you return to the cockpit after a layoff, not only will your performance snap back sooner to the levels you expect, but you'll have a leg up on injury prevention.

Notes on kayaking wouldn't be complete without a discussion about the indisputable and well documented value of good equipment. Your kayak should be specifically engineered to handle the maneuvers you intend to put it through. And, of course, your bootie needs to fit the seat and your legs need to fit the cockpit. Make sure your sprayskirt fits tightly so that you don't fill your kayak with water as you rock and roll. A swamped kayak is impossible to maneuver. Also, your sprayskirt must have a high-quality emergency release system, in case you have to pop it in a hurry. You should wear footwear designed for paddle sports. These high-tech shoes fit comfortably, have reinforced heel cups where the pressure on your foot is most intense, and are snugly sealed at the ankles. (You don't want a nasty hydraulic to suck your shoes off!) The shoes should be designed to drain any water that soaks in so that you don't paddle all day with water trapped around your feet. And finally, the soles should be tough so that you can hike any distance over any terrain to port your kayak from your car to the water. And as a last note, don't even think about snapping into the cockpit without a life jacket and helmet.

See you at the bottom of the rapids!

Martial Arts

To Strengthen:	Upper Legs, Hips, and Trunk	1–15
	Shoulders	16–25
	Neck	26
	Arms, Elbows, Wrists, and Hands	27–30
	Lower Legs, Ankles, and Feet	31–35

Coaches' Notes

In recent years, we have seen a renewed interest in martial arts among our clients. Their enthusiasm is fueled by media superstars who slash their way across television and movie screens with perfect bodies, heroic courage, uncompromising virtue, and impenetrable serenity. To people who seek physical perfection and the keys to life's mysteries, martial artists represent a compelling package. More than once, we've had to tone down an enthusiastic client by pointing out that these martial artists look good on the screen, but they got there by sweating in the dojo for years. And here's the kicker (pun intended): Their workouts are centered around offensive and defensive fighting.

Is the word "martial" (meaning "of or pertaining to war") a dead give-away? Hello. We will tell you what we tell our clients who ask our opinion. If you want to be a martial artist, it takes years of hard work and it can be painful. Someone somewhere is going to kick you.

Before you accuse us of complete insensitivity toward the beautiful philosophies and disciplines of martial arts, please know that we are fully aware and (mostly) supportive. We spend a great deal of time in Asia, working with athletes and dancers, and we incorporate aspects of Asian culture into our own practice. But we are fitness professionals who are devoted to building and maintaining the bodies of athletes. It is very difficult for us to deal with combat, where one person strikes another (even accidentally). It ruins our hard work. We never discourage an athlete from pursuing martial arts, but we prefer to focus our support on the broad disciplines of the training, rather than the specifics of fighting: grappling (judo and jujitsu) or contact (karate-do).

Although martial arts vary widely, they are all bound by the fact that they are excellent methods for achieving fitness. They all require agility, endurance, coordination, balance, strength, flexibility, and intelligence. Training begins with a great master (a teacher, or *sensei*, with no less than black belt) and the best protective equipment (as much as you can wear). Training is sequential and methodical, starting with the basics and progressing to advanced practice in each technique. The defined phases of learning a technique are kata (learning the technique), randori (free practice), and kumite (advanced practice). Each phase has three stages: warm-up, technique practice, and cool-down. You don't progress to a higher level until you have command of the lower one, and you learn to defend before you learn to attack. The net effect is a logical, careful progression toward mastery. And there's more. Martial arts train not only the body, but the total person. The discipline includes such Asian values as politeness, fraternity, serenity, modesty, seriousness, courage, formality, and integrity. Without question, the training—for both body and soul—is spectacular.

Injuries are inherent in contact sports, and the martial arts are no exception. Surprisingly, however, judo studies reveal an incidence of significant injury—one that will bench an athlete for more than twenty-four hours—of only 10 percent. To put this injury rate into context, it is below football or hockey and equal to wrestling. Karate-do does not fare so well, with a rate of 50 percent. The disparities in injury rates reflect the differences in the two sports. Trauma accounts for most of the injuries in both. Martial arts experts point out that the risk of traumatic injury is lessened when the competitors are skilled in technique, are evenly matched, use appropriate force, are sufficiently fit, wear protective equipment, fight in a regulated facility, and fight under the supervision of a qualified master.

If you are not able to compete and practice year-round, experts urge that you maintain your fitness base in the off-season with flexibility, strength, and cardiovascular work. And we would like to remind you that, once you've trained your body into a lean, mean (yet polite and serene) fighting machine, you need to be vigilant in protecting it. When we say that you should get a kick out of being totally fit, we don't mean it literally.

Pole Vault

To Strengthen:	Upper Legs, Hips, and Trunk	1–15
	Shoulders	16–25
	Neck	26
	Arms, Elbows, Wrists, and Hands	27–30
	Lower Legs, Ankles, and Feet	31–35

Coaches' Notes

Pole vaulting is a sport so ancient that we can scarcely trace its origin. It's possible that the first pole vaulter was a hunter who figured out how to cross a wide stream by running up to the bank, planting the tip of his wooden spear in the stream-bottom beneath the water, hoisting himself high up onto the shaft, and using the momentum of his run to catapult himself over the stream until his feet hit the opposite bank. Today, the stream is gone and the wooden spear has been replaced by an 18-foot Fiberglas® pole, but the principles are the same. And so are the results: a high-flying athlete and a heart-stopping moment, followed by the sweet relief of a successful landing.

Interestingly, a vaulter in training is taught that he or she is first and foremost a sprinter. It's necessary to define the athlete this way because the ability to sprint—make a searing, all-out approach to the bar—is a critical component in the vault, no less important than the ability to plant the pole. If the approach is uneven or too slow, the vaulter doesn't have the force necessary to get the pole into the vertical position. Bad ride. The athlete will end up on his or her bootie back down the runway.

Assuming that the approach is going to be a good one, the anatomy of a vault goes something like this: You begin by holding the pole to one side, supporting the weight in a grip wider than shoulder width. The pole should be angled up 15 to 20 degrees, with the tip higher than your head. Now, run. Smoothly, evenly, and fast. At the last stride, you move the pole up over your head with your arms separated. You bring the tip down and plant it in the box. Your top hand pulls down. Your bottom hand pushes up. Continue to press forward, bowing the pole. Hang on, now. When the pole has reached its maximum coil, it releases its energy—rebounds—to catapult you over the bar. When your pole is directly vertical, you will notice that the bar is still higher than you are. No problem. You continue your ascent with a gymnastic handstand and clear the bar in a neat jackknife. Back first, you relax and aim for landing. Did we mention a world's record?

Injuries in pole vaulting tend to be those common to all sprinters (see page 161). But there's more. (You didn't think the only dangerous aspect of the sport was the charge down the runway, did you?) Vaulters also risk damage to their shoulders during takeoffs and their back during landings. The good news comes from medical statisticians: most injuries to vaulters are caused by mistakes in planting the tip of the pole, so they are largely preventable with proper technique and preparation.

Training for the pole vault is a fine combination of all that we hold dear: cardiovascular work for sprinting, strength, and flexibility. None is more important than another, but of particular interest is flexibility. You have to be able to arch your back with your arms down as you clear the bar—not an easy maneuver, but necessary to keep you from hitting the bar with your chest, torqueing, and straining every muscle from your neck to your knees as you struggle to effect a landing. Additionally, flexibility allows you to relax into the landing and absorb the shock of impact on the mat. The ability to stay loose while still in full control goes a long way toward injury prevention, not to mention the fact that you look better.

Race Walking

To Strengthen:	Upper Legs, Hips, and Trunk	1–15
	Shoulders	16–25
	Lower Legs, Ankles, and Feet	31–35

Coaches' Notes

We were once consulted by an injured runner whose orthopedist had just ordered him to take a short layoff. We use the word "ordered" because the injury—a tibial stress fracture—was serious, and the prescription for rest was emphatically nonnegotiable. Like every runner we've ever known to be ordered out of his running shoes, this runner was grief-stricken and frantic to get back out onto the road so that he would not lose his training base. He came to us to discuss emergency options: other activities or modified activities that would approximate the cardiovascular and biomechanical benefits of running, but without the pounding. He had given the matter considerable thought on his way over and had logically concluded that race walking would be a good alternative to running, especially if he did it late at night when no one would see him swinging his hips down the road. He noted rather sheepishly that it "looks prissy," but it moves an athlete forward and does not appear to be hard on the body. So, what did we think? We cracked up. After we explained the mechanics of race walking, our client opted to put on a float belt, "run" suspended in the deep end of a swimming pool, and leave the "prissy" sport to athletes who can take a real beating.

The misconceptions about race walking held by our running friend are universal. The first time people see a race walker, their impressions are that "it looks prissy," it's just fast walking, and it can't be all that tough. These impressions last until a Wharton assures them otherwise, or they try race walking for themselves. Either way, a second look at race walking gives a whole new respect for the sport.

Race walking is distinguished from "running" in that there is no airborne phase in the gait. In other words, one foot is always on the ground. You can't lift your rear foot and bring it into a step until your front foot is firmly in contact with the surface. Race walking is distinguished from "walking" in that the whole time your foot is on the ground, the knee of that leg has to be straight. The strain on that leg is enormous as you move your body forward, over the foot on the ground, with as long a stride as possible. While you're moving over the grounded foot, your rear foot is straining to stay on the ground until the stride is completed. Only then can your rear foot break contact. This phase requires extreme flexibility of your foot and ankle, and places great stress on the back of your leg. Like a sprinter, you close your fists and pump with your arms to achieve momentum by amplifying the action of your lower body. Unlike a sprinter, however, you are restricted to a completely upright posture. No leaning forward is allowed. It's one of the real challenges of the sport. This is in direct contrast to the physics of walking as we understand it. Walking has been described as controlled falling. Essentially, you lean forward until you are about to fall and, at the last possible moment, you stick out one foot to catch yourself. This is a step. Balance on that one foot and lean forward until you start to fall and then catch yourself with the other foot. And so on. The more far forward you lean and the more aggressive your "catch," the faster you walk until you are going so fast that you anticipate the fall and prepare for it by picking up your back foot before you've passed your torso over the front foot. When both feet are off the ground at the same time, you've entered the airborne phase. This is "running." So how do you achieve speed when you can neither lean forward nor get airborne? The hip swing. By using that turbocharge at the hip, you get that slight forward thrust for momentum. It literally pops your back leg forward.

Injuries in race walking are generally of the lower extremities: muscles along the tibia tend to strain if the ankles and feet are inflexible, and the athlete has difficulty in keeping the rear foot on the ground. (Now you see why we discouraged race walking as an alternative for our runner with the tibial stress fracture.) The extreme trunk rotation places an athlete at risk for strains in the lower back and abdominal muscle groups. And the straight-leg technique, as we said, places great strain on the back of the leg—specifically, the Achilles tendon, the gastrocs, and posterior knee. Injury prevention is a function of strength and flexibility training combined with good technique. Supplemental training should include upper body work.

Race walking is more well known in Europe than in the United States, but it's gaining in popularity as athletes become familiar with its distinctive gait and impressive fitness benefits.

Racquetball

To Strengthen:	Upper Legs, Hips, and Trunk	1–15
	Shoulders	16–25
	Neck	26
	Arms, Elbows, Wrists, and Hands	27–30
	Lower Legs, Ankles, and Feet	31–35

Coaches' Notes

A couple of years ago, we were consulted to design a rehab program for a racquetball player—a ranked national champion with an arm of gold, a meteoric career, and a mysterious injury. She came into our clinic on crutches, with her foot in a cast. In evaluating her, we had to have the facts, so we asked, "What's broken and how did it happen?" She was clearly embarrassed as she muttered and stammered, "Uh, I broke a couple of . . . um . . . toes." OK. No big deal. That happens in racquetball. Had she hit the wall? "No." Had another player stepped on her? "No." Had she dropped the racquet on her foot? "No." We were running out of scenarios to suggest. Exasperated, we asked, "You broke your toes standing in the middle of the floor all by yourself, without falling, without hitting the wall, and without dropping anything?!?" She rolled her eyes and nodded her head. We had finally gotten the picture. And suddenly we knew what she had done. She had been running forward in shoes that were laced too loosely. Her feet were not snug. She had stopped suddenly to back up for a shot. Well, at least her shoe had stopped. Her foot had slid forward and slammed into the front of her shoe, fracturing a couple of toes. Jim calls it "Toe Jam," and it happens occasionally in court sports that require ballistic direction changes. We use this anecdote about our embarrassed champion to demonstrate that racquetball can be a contact sport, even when there's no one else around.

Racquetball is a quick game. Little time is spent standing around the court, waiting for the next move. That's what we like about it. It's quick because of a small lightweight racquet, a lightning-fast rubber ball, and a small enclosed space. But those features that give it all the components of a good workout also make it inherently dangerous. The racquet, because it is so small, does not slow the arm or wrist down (as a tennis racquet would). The game is played with rapid snaps and slaps that can be easily out of control and can violently wrench a joint. Additionally, because the racquet is light, the athlete might not ever build strength sufficient to sustain a difficult game. And finally, because the action is so rapid, collisions with the wall and other players are real possibilities when things get heated up on the court. In fact, the most dangerous injury in racquetball is getting hit in the eye with a racquet or the ball.

Overuse injuries are common in racquetball. Some players are plagued by racquetball versions of "tennis elbow"—valgus overload syndrome or medial epicondylitis—that usually flare with badly executed forehand shots for which the body is not prepared. Additionally, we see tendinitis in the wrist. The bad news is that overuse injuries are not left behind on the court. They tend to follow a player into everyday life, nagging him or her throughout the accomplishment of seemingly simple tasks such as opening jars or turning ignition keys. The good news is that overuse injuries are frequently healed by active rehabilitation that does not include surgery. And the even better news is that overuse injuries are largely preventable with good training that includes strength and flexibility.

Racquetball is a wonderful workout. When played hard, regularly (four times a week), and for at least 45 minutes per game, it can provide a fine cardiovascular workout. Supplemental strength and flexibility work are musts, to give you maximum control during the game and prevent injuries. Remember to warm up before you get onto the court.

A final word: Wear eye protection (with lenses) specifically made for racquet sports. Studies have concluded that your own glasses—even if they're shatterproof—provide NO effective protection on the court and are, in fact, dangerous. Also, we caution you to snugly lace and tie those shoes!

Rock Climbing

To Strengthen:	Upper Legs, Hips, and Trunk	1–15
	Shoulders	16–25
	Neck	26
	Arms, Elbows, Wrists, and Hands	27–30
	Lower Legs, Ankles, and Feet	31–35

Coaches' Notes

Rock climbing is a sport that no longer requires a rock. All it requires is a climb. Where there's a wall, there's a way. Almost. (It helps if the wall has been engineered with ledges for toeholds and crevices for finger grips.) From fitness centers in Manhattan to office suites in San Francisco, the great outdoors is being plastered into recreational space for people who enjoy "climbing the walls."

If you are going to climb, starting indoors on one of these simulated vertical faces can be a good way to train safely. The indoor wall will present you with technical challenges, but without loose gravel, hidden scorpions, razor-sharp cracks, slippery moss, searing heat, freezing snow, driving rain, or sudden sunsets. It's a chance to hone your basic skills before you have to experience the true "nature" of the sport. (As one of our friends bluntly noted, "Nature is a little messy.") In fact, many climbers never even bother to take the activity outside. Climbing is fun, no matter where you tie on.

Rock climbing is a sport for people of all sizes. We learned this as we watched a tiny woman defy gravity. She crawled up a sheer cliff like Spider Woman until she encountered an overhang. We assumed that the climb was certainly concluded, but we assumed wrong. She reached out back over her head and then edged upside down and horizontally across the underside of the rock until she rounded a lip, emerged, and continued the climb vertically. When we remarked about her diminutive size, the instructor who was providing commentary pointed out that she was as strong as she needed to be to support her own weight. The bigger the climber, the stronger he or she needs to be.

Unique among athletes, rock climbers have to have strength in their fingers and toes to match the strength in their bodies. If you can't grip with your fingers or wedge with your toes, it makes little difference that you are fit everywhere else. Total strength is critically important. Equally important is flexibility, which gives you the ability to take advantage of a full range of motion, to span a great distance, to control your body, and to recover fully and quickly from a maneuver. And the final component for success in climbing is stamina. You don't want to get up the wall and discover that you're too exhausted to climb down. Remember, what (and who) goes up must come down, and *you* should decide when and how. The climb itself will not provide an amazing cardiovascular workout. Even if it did provide a good workout, most climbers do it too infrequently for it to be considered effective. You'll have to supplement your fitness program with some cardio work—running, swimming, or cycling four to five times per week at 45 minutes per session—to increase your endurance and give you an added boost when you take your climbing to altitude.

Not surprisingly, injuries in climbing are relatively few. And most are in the hand—specifically, the ring finger and the tendons that lead to it. This small area takes the greatest stress when a climber grips a ledge and then lifts his or her body from the hand. Other common injuries are related to cuts, scrapes, rope burns, pinches, and bruises from slipping. The ultimate horror of every beginning climber—and most experienced ones—is falling. Although unquestionably dangerous, falling does not automatically constitute a fatal accident when safety equipment is used and safety procedures are in place.

Training and skill go a long way in preventing injury, but equipment may be even more important. Rock climbing gear takes a beating with every adventure, so you will want to maintain yours as if your life depended on it—it does! Inspect your gear before and after every climb. If you see any wear and tear, either repair or replace it immediately. Take no chances with trying to get "one more climb" out of it. And make certain that your shoes are in great shape.

Work with the best instructors you can find. Climb only with the most skilled and reliable companions. Climb only when you feel ready. Be warmed up, rested, hydrated, and fueled to make every climb your best. Today, if you say, "I'm climbing the walls!" it no longer means that you're going crazy. It means that you're getting fit. That's about as sane as you can get.

Rowing/Sculling

To Strengthen:	Upper Legs, Hips, and Trunk	1–15
	Shoulders	16–25
	Neck	26
	Arms, Elbows, Wrists, and Hands	27–30
	Lower Legs, Ankles, and Feet	31–35

Coaches' Notes

We work with Reid Boates, a good friend who, when he wants us to accomplish more than our usual miracles, gives us our assignment and then says, "Row well and live." Death threats notwithstanding, we are amused by the metaphor of getting a job done by working away at it one stroke at a time, as if life depended on it (in a galley slave kind of way). It's this methodical progression toward a goal that we find so attractive about rowing and sculling. The sports require patience and repetitive effort, but surely and eventually they'll get you wherever you're going. Guaranteed. And there is something deeply satisfying in that.

You row with one oar and scull with two, but the biomechanics and physical demands of the two sports are very similar, so we'll discuss them together. Essentially, you sit with your arms extended in front of you and the oar grasped in your hands. You put the tip of the oar into the water and then pull the handle toward you, pressing against the resistance of the water and propelling your craft. When you arrive at the end of the stroke, you lift the tip of the oar out of the water, return to the beginning position of the stroke, reinsert the tip into the water, and stroke again. Your back is straight, but you flex (bend) at the hips to assist your arms in moving the oar forward, and you extend (straighten out) to assist in moving the paddle backward. Your feet, braced in footrests, are used to transmit power through your whole body as you roll your seat fore and aft. If technique is the craft, then power and rhythm are the art. True mastery comes in knowing how far into the water you plunge the tip of the oar, how hard to pull against the resistance of the water, and how fast to initiate the stroke. And the next. And the next . . . .

Because rowing and sculling are the ultimate repetitive-action sports, it only makes sense that repetitive injuries would be the plague of the athletes. And, although we think of how the sport places stress on those powerfully working arms and shoulders, most of the injuries are in the knees. It makes sense. The athlete is locked into a tightly constricted position, extending and flexing, pulling and pushing with knees in a very rigid back-and-forth path. The joints get irritated. Injuries of the lower back are also common. The reasons are the same: specific, constricted tracking with extension and flexion over and over until irritation sets in. Back difficulties are exacerbated by pressure from sitting on and pushing against the hard seat. Also, especially in competitive training and rowing, the strain to the back can be so extreme that an athlete can actually stress-fracture his or her ribs. So much for "Row, row, row your boat GENTLY down the stream . . . ."

We also want to caution coxswains against occupational hazards that plague the loud and annoying. Olympic Games historians report that, in Amsterdam in 1928, "The U.S. was represented by the crew from the University of California at Berkeley. *New York Times* correspondent Wythe Williams described [the calls of] coxswain Don Blessing as 'one of the greatest performances of demoniacal howling ever heard on a territorial planet. . . . He gave the impression of a terrier suddenly gone mad.' But such language and what a vocabulary! After they had won the Olympic championship, the galley slaves, following the custom, grabbed their tormentor and threw him into the middle of the Sloten Canal."* Let this serve as a warning to us all.

Rowing and sculling are wonderful exercise, but they aren't perfect by a long shot. Because the tracking of your body is so specific, you're likely to have serious muscle imbalances if you don't supplement your program with a comprehensive strength program. Also, flexibility is critical in holding off the repetitive stress injuries unfortunately inherent in these sports. Having a full range of motion in joints—specifically, hips, knees, shoulders, wrists, and back—will help keep you free from irritations and nerve impingements. And finally, you'll want to add a good cardiovascular program to your workout. Stamina goes a long way toward winning. Warm up before you step into the boat, particularly if the day is cold. Remember to take in plenty of fluids, even on cold days. And have fun. As our friend Reid says, "Row well and live!"

Rugby

To Strengthen:	Upper Legs, Hips, and Trunk	1–15
	Shoulders	16–25
	Neck	26
	Arms, Elbows, Wrists, and Hands	27–30
	Lower Legs, Ankles, and Feet	31–35

Coaches' Notes

Rugby enjoys the reputation of being one of the most brutal sports in the world. Yet, in spite of its blood-and-guts image, international medical statistical studies indicate that rugby is a relatively safe sport. We have seen rugby played, so we have to seriously question the statistics. We suggest they may be skewed by rugby players' perceptions regarding "serious" injury and their collective ability (or inability) to judge a medical situation. We have a rugby-loving friend who tells of witnessing a bad hit during a rugby match, leaping from the sidelines, plunging into the pandemonium, and asking, "Is Ramon OK?" The answer was, "Oh, yeah. He's OK. We're just going to stick this bone back through the skin, and he's going right back in. Right, Ramon?" So much for statistics.

As far as we can tell, "rugby" may very well be synonymous with "injury." One British study reported that most rugby injuries are cuts (40 percent). Cuts are followed by muscle and tendon injuries (22 percent),

The Complete Book of the Olympics by David Wallechinsky. (1991). Little, Brown & Company: Canada.

and injuries to joints (21 percent), heads (6.5 percent), bones (6 percent), and, finally, "other." Danger is everywhere. As a scrum collapses (and it often does), struggling players are knotted into a dangerous human macramé. A player in the wrong place at the wrong time can get crushed under the pressing weight of the straining teams. Tackles are thrown by hard-charging players wearing no protective equipment. The risk of injury is as great to the tacklers as it is to the tackled. Mauls, rucks, and pileups speak for themselves. Here, legs, knees, and feet take beatings. Even in lineouts, where no contact should take place, players suffer trauma to joints from the sudden stopping and starting, accidental collisions, and deliberate (frequent and illegal!) interference that happens so fast that a referee can't catch it.

Injury prevention is a matter of selecting another, kinder, gentler sport. But we know you aren't going to do that, so we'll tell you that rugby statistics reveal something interesting: the more fit the player, the less likely he or she is to be injured. The conclusion you should draw is that you need to get yourself to the gym immediately. Not only will you play better, but you'll be more likely to finish the game in one piece. In addition, rugby coaching experts say you should always wear a mouth guard to protect your teeth, and, more important, to lessen your risk of concussion by providing a barrier between an opponent's boot and your temporomandibular joint.

Rugby is good exercise, but, if you're like most players, you aren't able to play more than once a week, so you can't count on it to provide your total fitness program. Because rugby is arguably one of the most demanding sports on the field, you need to be strong and flexible and to have enough stamina to maintain energy and control throughout the game. Again, you need to pay attention to the statistics that highlight the link between fitness and injury prevention. To be a good player, you need to supplement your playing time with time in the gym. And you need to build a solid cardiovascular program with running, cycling, or swimming. Play hard, but be smart.

Running

To Strengthen:	Upper Legs, Hips, and Trunk	1–15
	Shoulders	16–25
	Lower Legs, Ankles, and Feet	31–35

Coaches' Notes

Occasionally, we will get a new client who says, "I want to lose weight so I've decided to take up running." We say, tell that to your feet. If you knew that running causes your feet to hit the ground at forces 1.5 to 5 times your present body weight, and that each foot hits the ground 100 times per mile and over 5,000 times per hour, would you still take up running while you're heavy? Or would you try to lighten your load just a little *before* you place all that stress on your feet? It's a conundrum, to be certain. But no matter how much you weigh, running can do wonderful things for your body and soul. Not only is running an important component of many other sports, but it stands alone as an efficient, effective cardiovascular workout that slips easily into a jam-packed schedule.

Running begins as walking. Left. Right. Left. Right. As you accelerate, eventually you move so fast that you automatically advance to an airborne phase with both feet off the ground at the same time. This single moment simply expresses the basic difference between walking and running. The actual mechanics of running are miracles in shock absorption and energy transfer. When your front heel strikes the ground, and you pass your torso over the top of it, your foot begins to "load"— it takes your weight. Your shin (tibia) rotates slightly to the inside. Your loading foot (at first in supination with ankle angled, pointing the sole of the foot to the inside) flattens under the pressure of your weight, and then, when it has reached its maximum compression (now in pronation with ankle angled, pointing the sole of the foot to the outside), tendons and muscles recoil like a spring to restore your foot to its neutral (supinated) position, giving you a boost up and forward. Another way to visualize this is to picture your arch flattening out and then springing back into shape as you roll your weight from your heel onto the ball of your foot. Experts describe this as "vertical-to-longitudinal torque conversion." While your loading foot is doing its work, your rear foot is coming up and around in a cyclical pattern to take its place. But your feet and legs are not working alone. All major muscle groups demonstrate significant increases in activity. Indeed, running engages the entire body.

The benefits are not only muscular. We consider the cardiovascular function gained in running to be even more significant. Runners tell a story about a man who had "let himself go." He had deteriorated into such poor health that he had no hope for recovery. His life was miserable. He smoked. He ate badly. He was confined to a sagging recliner in front of his TV. He could barely function. One day he decided that, because he couldn't endure his debilitation any longer, he would "end it all" by running out the front door and across his lawn where he would surely drop dead from the inevitable heart attack. So he hoisted his obese body out of his recliner, wept, "Good-bye, cruel world!" and lurched out the front door. He ran until he dropped. But he didn't die. He lay there until he could catch his breath and then walked back into the house, determined to try it again the next day. Oddly, however, he felt a little better. (Runners love to hear this part of the story; they start to wink and nudge each other when it's told.) The next day, the sickly man repeated the suicide attempt. This time he got a little farther across the lawn before he collapsed. But again, he didn't die. And, oddly, he felt even better. (Runners usually start to quietly weep here.) Every day the man tried to kill himself and every day he failed, but he got farther and farther across the lawn each time. Soon, his weight returned to normal, his energy picked up, and his general health improved. He quit smoking and started eating better. He turned off the TV and got out of his recliner more. He became a runner and was saved. (At this point in the telling of the story, runners generally cheer, leap up, and high-five each other.) The story might be exaggerated, and we don't recommend you fling yourself into running without checking with your doctor, but most runners will tell you a personal tale of redemption, and most of them will cite cardiovascular benefits—the heart attack that DIDN'T happen—as the greatest plus of the sport. Getting cardiovascularly fit is a simple matter of gradually stressing your system until it responds by getting stronger. As it learns to work, your heart becomes more efficient. Lung function is increased. Blood circulates and is oxygenated more efficiently. Toxins are flushed. Running turns up the heat and revs up your metabolism. As you become more fit and begin to burn body fat more efficiently, formerly alarming blood chemistries often start to come into normal ranges. Cholesterol levels often drop. (Atlanta running coach Roy Benson calls this "becoming a better butter burner.") Glowing good health is on the way!

Running, in spite of all its benefits, is also a sport in which injuries are common. It is, of course, the ultimate repetitive activity. Sports medicine experts classify injuries into two categories: those that are caused by circumstances and those that are caused by the runner's physiology. Of those that are caused by circumstances, training mistakes—running too much, too soon, and too often—lead the list. Of those injuries caused by a runner's physiology, imbalance, misalignment, and inflexibility are the most common. No matter what the cause of the problem, running tends to be fairly unforgiving. Small things make big differences when they're multiplied and amplified to the extent that running demands. Everything has to work. And, equally important, everything has to work together. Breakdowns can occur in perfectly healthy places when the failure is actually somewhere else up or down the line. For example, a weak hamstring that cannot do its job might force compensations all the way down the leg, and show up as pain and dysfunction in the Achilles tendon—nearly forty inches below the "real" problem. A weakened lower back may cause a slight pelvic list on one side that will drop one leg low and cause the foot to hit the ground a nanosecond before it should. The result could be knee and ankle pain, and a slight limp. The runner, concluding that a "leg length discrepancy" is the culprit, might slip a lift into the heel of the other shoe. Now the imbalance is even greater and triggers a domino effect of cascading injuries.

You will want to supplement your running program with strength training—particularly for the upper body—and flexibility work, to offset the hammering and limited range of motion your body takes in the repetitive, forward tracking of a running gait.

Our advice to all runners is to pay attention to your bodies. Buy the best shoes you can afford and select them under the guidance of an experienced, trusted person. Start your running program slowly, and increment your mileage and the intensity of your workouts gradually. If injury strikes, seek advice from a physician who treats runners and running injuries. And, once you get that advice, heed it. Be smart and you'll live to run another day.

A final word: *please* hydrate adequately before, during, and after your workout. If you feel thirsty, you have already begun to dehydrate. Electrolyte replacement fluids—sports drinks—are great, but water is just fine for most programs. Our experts tell us that the colder the fluid, the better.

Running—Marathon

| To Strengthen: | Upper Legs, Hips, and Trunk | 1–15 |
| | Lower Legs, Ankles, and Feet | 31–35 |

Coaches' Notes

When we train beginning distance runners, one of the first questions we're asked is: "Why is the marathon such a peculiar distance? Why is it 26 miles *AND* 385 yards?" It always amuses us that the overwhelming focus of concern is that pesky 385 yards. If we were asking the questions, we would demand to know more about that 26 miles. Let us give you a quick marathon history lesson. No one knows the exact details of the origin, but it is generally accepted that the marathon commemorates Phidippides, an overly enthusiastic Greek messenger who ran 25 miles—from the plains of Marathon to Athens—to bring news of the victory of the Athenians against Darius the Great in 490 BC. Phidippides arrived in Athens, shouted, "Rejoice! We conquer!" and dropped over dead. Now, that should have been the end of it, but some runner took a look at the Phidippides incident and said, "Whoa! Killed him! Let's make a sport out of it and do it competitively!" And, it must have sounded good to the athletes who subscribed to the "More is Better" school of running, because it caught on. The original 25 miles were a long way to run, but evidently not quite long enough because, in 1908, at the London Olympic Games, King Edward VII's youngest daughter decided that she wanted to see the start of the marathon from her throne at White City Stadium, although accommodating this little princess meant adding a couple of miles to the course. Royal request became royal decree. No one thought of moving the kid's throne out onto the course. No. They just added the miles. And, when it was over, no one thought of removing those additional miles for the following Olympiad. No. They kept them in. Hence, today's marathon is set at 26.2 miles and is embraced by the running community as the ultimate challenge.

To understand the marathon, it is necessary to restate the obvious: 26.2 miles is a *long* way to run. Consequently, you train to be as efficient as possible by designing a running style that maximizes your body's use of fuel and hydration, and conserves your energy for the long haul. It's a delicate balancing act that requires a gradual adaptation to distance and a lot of practice to "work out the bugs." Although speed is eventually important to competitive runners, even they will tell you that they worried about conquering the *distance* first. Successful pacing in the marathon means that you run as fast as you can, but you reserve enough energy to get you to the finish line—and one important inch beyond it. The marathon gait is distinguished from shorter-distance gaits by adaptations designed to keep you moving forward while expending as little energy as possible: a more upright posture in your torso, a shorter stride, a lower knee lift, relaxed arms carried lower, and open hands. The net effect is efficiency.

High mileage and overuse injuries go hand in hand, unfortunately. We once asked a friend how she happened to know so much about physiology. She replied, "Are you kidding? I'm a marathon runner! At one time or another, I've torn up EVERY bone, muscle, ligament, and tendon in my entire body. I merely carry the broken part into the physiatrist's office, and ask, 'What is this, where did it used to go, what did it used to do, and how can I get it all back together again?' Over the years, I've learned so much!" We all laughed. But her points are well taken. First, injury is the companion of marathon runners. And second, the training teaches you about your own body, piece by piece. There is much you can do to mitigate the risks. Train smart.

Running—especially high-mileage running—hammers your musculoskeletal system. This is the first part of a natural cycle of strength building. When you stress muscles, bones, and attachments, tissues break down. But if you give them time, the tissues repair themselves and make one important adaptation: they come back even stronger. Then you go out and hammer them again, breaking them back down. And the cycle is repeated. Each time, the tissues repair more strongly, and you become a better runner. All successful runners eventually discover the balance: knowing how much to stress the body during the run, and how long to allow the body to remodel itself after the damage you inflict. You learn by hitting the trail, keeping written mileage and performance records, and paying close attention to how you feel. We call it "Trail and Error." Hopefully, you'll have a lot of "Trail" and very little "Error." Perfect your technique during short distances and then work up to longer distances very gradually. Sudden increases in mileage can be hazardous to your health.

Another risk in marathon running is that, unlike most other running events, it is ALWAYS off track. This means that you will have to contend with uneven surfaces, unmeasured distances, potholes, debris, big dogs with attitude, engine exhaust from badly tuned cars, and a host of other inconveniences. It's all part of the fun of the sport, but it does mean that you must be vigilant.

Marathon running is, without question, a superior cardiovascular workout, but not a well-rounded fitness program. You will want to supplement your workout with strength training—particularly in your upper body. By the way, you'll be surprised at the improvement in your running performance when you strengthen your upper body. As you fatigue during the marathon, you tend to lean forward, leading your body with your chin. (This is a nice way to say that you "droop.") As your chin heads south, your chest compresses and your ability to take a deep breath is impeded. Also, your body starts to struggle to keep you upright by recruiting assistance from other muscles. Fighting fatigue causes even more fatigue. A strong upper body stops trouble in its tracks. Besides strength training, you will want to have a good flexibility program. Running is repetitive and puts your body on a very narrow track. Flexibility opens up ranges of motion on joints that are really constricted. Additionally, flexibility—the ability to move freely—will speed recovery from the hammering you take when you run by helping you flush metabolic waste from your muscles and recruit oxygen-carrying blood flow to assist healing.

A final word: One of the most important components in marathon training, and one of the least observed, is REST. You are tearing down your body when you hit high mileage, and you need to give it time to recover. Overtraining can lead to a wide variety of serious physical and emotional difficulties. A day off is NOT a day wasted. It's a day of recovering, rebuilding, replenishing, and refreshing.

Running—Sprinting

Coaches' Notes

If there was ever a sport that could keep you on your toes, this is it. Olympic champion sprinter Jesse Owens once disclosed the secret of his success when he told a London reporter, "I let my feet spend as little time on the ground as possible. From the air, fast down, and from the ground, fast up. My foot is only a fraction of the time on the track." The gait in "normal" running is: strike the ground with your heel, roll up over the ball of your foot to your toes, push off, lift your foot up, extend it out, and repeat. Sprinting distinguishes itself from this gait by commanding a strike with the ball of your foot. In other words, instead of a heel-toe-heel-toe cadence, sprinting is toe-toe-toe-toe. And, of course, it is faster. In fact, you leave the blocks as though you have been shot from a cannon—an acceleration process that is more miraculous than you can imagine. This explosive power is marshaled and harnessed as you crouch in the blocks and preload your muscles—specifically, powerful quadriceps. You store tension so that when you choose finally to release, or when the starter's shot begins a race, the release is ballistic. But the real miracle occurs in your upper body. By closing your fists and swinging your arms, you amplify the capability of your legs. Sports medicine experts call it "crossed-extensor reciprocal eccentric and concentric energy utilization." Translation: By loading tension into your left hand and swinging your left arm in direct opposition to your right leg, you create a sort of total anatomical "partnership" far more powerful than the sum of your parts. If you doubt it, try sprinting with your arms down. You'll be stunned by the immediate and total deterioration of your form and speed.

Sprinting may be miraculous, but it is also incredibly hard on your body. Injuries unfortunately are all too common. Not only must the entire body be strong, but it must be flexible. The 1960 Olympic gold medalist in the 100 meter sprint, Armin Hary, noted that his famous ballistic start was more than just quick reflexes. He said, "More important to me is the fact that I have learned, through relaxation, how to achieve full stride and smooth forward action very early in the race." Sprinters need full range of motion in all joints. Remember that little things make big differences in running. Small investments in training yield huge dividends. Conversely, small mistakes are amplified into massive injuries. This is especially true of sprinting where the pounding is enormous, the racing flats are thin, the stakes are high, and the speed is "all out." Overuse injuries lead the list of injuries. Of course.

One of the interesting occupational hazards of sprinters is the track itself. Running on a banked track in the signature counterclockwise direction can profoundly stress the joints from the hips to the feet. The inside foot is forced into supination—that is, the outside edge of the foot is angled down, and the arch side of the foot is angled up. And the outside foot is forced into the opposite position. We recommend a serious flexibility initiative to protect your joints, and we advise you to take a few laps in the opposite direction during every workout. When you do this, make sure the track is cleared of other runners before you whip around and run the other way. Nothing is harder to explain than a face-to-face collision on the track.

Shot Put

To Strengthen:	Upper Legs, Hips, and Trunk	1–15
	Shoulders	16–25
	Arms, Elbows, Wrists, and Hands	27–30
	Lower Legs, Ankles, and Feet	31–35

Coaches' Notes

Shot put is one of our favorite sports because it has its origins in antiquity. In fact, it has been in our repertory of games since 600 BC and has managed to maintain the simple elegance of its heritage. It is called "putting" the shot rather than "throwing" because the shot is too heavy (sixteen pounds) to hurl. It is tucked up under the chin and "pushed" into its trajectory. Or at least this is how it appears to the casual observer. As in all things simple and elegant, there is much more beneath the surface.

Athletes today use a winding preparation similar to that of a discus thrower. Although personal styles and techniques vary widely, the principles of torque are consistent. As you whirl, you produce momentum that allows you to transfer energy from your body to the shot's trajectory. The tricky part is to create powerful torque, maintain delicate balance, and engineer a successful thrust of the shot—all with a sixteen-pound weight mashed against one side of your neck. The forces of the torque are so brutal and the consequences of a misstep or fatigue are so damaging to the body that coaches recommend that practice be limited. This is one sport where practice does not make perfect. Practice makes problems. Get it right the first couple of times and hit the showers.

Knees, back, hips, shoulders, and wrists suffer the most injuries in early season and with new athletes. As the season progresses or the athlete becomes more proficient, hands and fingers are added to the list. Why? Because a more capable athlete will hold the shot higher in the hand and thrust the shot from the fingertips.

We advise our shot putters that, although this is a great sport, it does not provide a comprehensive fitness program. Of particular concern in training should be the imbalance inherent in handling a sixteen-pound shot on one side of your body. Weight training should be orchestrated to offset this enormous imbalance. Additionally, we recommend a good cardiovascular workout—running is our preference for you. And, of course, an Active-Isolated flexibility program is critical to give you a strong and controlled full range of motion in all muscles and joints.

As a final note, we caution you to be discriminating about your practice equipment. 1928 Olympic gold medalist John Kuck started his career in shot put when he was only four years old. He found a three-pound agate stone sphere in his front yard and started throwing it around for fun. Later, his family discovered that his "shot put" was a 20,000-year-old Native American relic!

Skating—Ice

To Strengthen:	Upper Legs, Hips, and Trunk	1–15
	Lower Legs, Ankles, and Feet	31–35
	If you speed skate or lift a partner, add:	
	Shoulders	16–25
	Arms, Elbows, Wrists, and Hands	27–30

Coaches' Notes

We were once consulted by an ice skater whose complaint was numb toes. Stunned by the obvious, we were tempted to say, "Hey, ice'll do that every time. Warm up, buddy. Slug down a hot toddy and call us in the morning." But we have been in sports too long to hear the word "numb" without some alarm. In this case, it was a good thing that we resisted the urge to take a glib approach. Indeed, this skater was experiencing loss of sensation because of nerve compression caused by skates that were too small and laced too tightly. In his case, fixing the problem was a simple matter of adjusting boots. Not all skaters are that lucky.

The sport of skating is as dangerous as any activity that combines high speed with slick, hard surfaces. And no one is immune. Levels of participation are as varied as the risks of injury. Recreational and beginning skaters are statistically more prone to trauma—hitting the ice. Competitive and advanced skaters experience more chronic and overuse injuries, such as stress fractures. At particular risk are feet, ankles, lower legs, knees, hips, groin, back, shoulders, elbows, wrists, and hands. Did the experts leave *anything* out??? When one examines the results of research on skating injuries, one becomes acutely aware that the hair might be the only safe spot on the body. (To be frank, we would not be at all shocked if we came across a journal article entitled "The Cold Truth About Hair Follicle Trauma in Skating.")

One aspect of our job as trainers is to study a sport microscopically and mitigate as many factors that contribute to injuries of our clients as possible. Unfortunately, one of the contributing factors in skating is cold weather, and our professional skaters have all taken a narrow-minded view of our recommendation to warm up the rink. Truthfully, we know there is nothing we can do to turn up the furnace, but the effects of cold on anatomy and physiology have been well documented, and sometimes just being aware of them can help. For example, muscles start to fire less effectively when their temperature is dropped by as few as two degrees. And aerobic capacity is decreased in direct proportion. Warming up muscles slowly before you step out onto the ice and wearing protective clothing might help give the muscles that needed edge against the cold. And the cold can be deceiving; it can trick you into thinking that you are cooler than you are. When your skin is cold, it's easy to forget that your core temperature is rising to meet the physical demands of the skating and to warm your muscles as they fire. In fact, when you work hard, you sweat even when the temperature drops below zero! It doesn't take long for dehydration to set in. In dehydration, blood volumes diminish, and muscles struggle for oxygen that is delivered less and less with every stroke of your heart. Additionally, cells in your muscles—once plumped up with water—are drying out and shriveling. Microtearing and damage set in. Your heart rate increases, trying to make up for the slack. Nothing works right. Fatigue sets in. You become less coordinated. And you lose the competition. Our message to you simply is to DRINK! Additionally, beware of cold injuries such as windburn and frostbite. Protect exposed body parts with clothing specifically designed to keep you warm, to wick perspiration out and block moisture from soaking in, to maximize your aerodynamics, and to "give" with every movement.

Skating is a wonderful aerobic workout and a fabulous lower body workout, but you will need to supplement your program with strength work on your upper body and Active-Isolated Stretching to ensure yourself a full range of motion. Pay particular attention to working feet and ankles that are locked into position and constricted in your boots.

Skating—In-Line

| To Strengthen: | Upper Legs, Hips, and Trunk | 1–15 |
| | Lower Legs, Ankles, and Feet | 31–35 |

Coaches' Notes

Because in-line skating is a relatively new sport, we have had the pleasure of watching it evolve—literally. Our clinic is near the west boundary of Central Park in New York, so, over the past few years, we have had a vantage point for viewing the never-ending parade of in-line skaters. At first, they were die-hard, off-season snow skiers who streaked through the park in summer with ski poles to keep in slope shape as they prayed for the rapid return of winter. Then we suffered through what we called the "Neon Phase," when color-coordinated, blindingly bright boots, wheels, sunglasses, and clothing were the rage. And now we're in the "Urban Guerrilla Phase"; more skaters appear to be sporting tattoos and attitude. No matter. Sport is sport is sport. It makes no difference what you wear, what your motivation is, or what attitude you assume. As long as you're out there, working out and having fun, Whartons are happy.

In-line skating is now designated as an "extreme" sport. It earned its reputation as "extreme" by combining speed, aerobatics, and acrobatics into gravity-defying choreography that can, at times, threaten life and limb. An athlete who takes the sport to the extreme is called an "aggro"—an "aggressive skater." Although we *all* have moments when we think of ourselves as aggros, most of us, most of the time, fall (no pun intended) into a range a little less aggro and a little more earth-bound. It is no wonder that in-line skating is enjoying such rampant popularity. It's fun and uncomplicated. To participate requires one skater, one pair of skates, protective equipment, and a stretch of pavement. (Unless you're an aggro. Then you need to add railing, steps, vaults, ramps, culverts, and an insurance agent with a sense of humor.)

Injuries that haunt in-line skaters are nearly identical to those that haunt ice skaters. Most injuries are traumatic: they occur when a skater falls or slams into something. Overuse and chronic injuries such as tendinitis are also common. Experts advise that injuries involving trauma can be mitigated with the use of protective equipment such as wrist and knee guards and the all-important helmet. Literature on in-line skating is loaded with admonishments to closely monitor the surface on which you skate. Look for holes, ridges, bumps, and debris. Be especially vigilant if you change the time of day (or night) when you skate, because light transforms the way surfaces look. A demon ridge that casts a long shadow at five o'clock in the afternoon may disappear altogether at high noon. And if you are skating in a group, be considerate. When you spot an obstacle, call it out for those who are skating behind you. Oh, yes, and skate around it.

Selecting the right skates is an important component to your success in the sport. We recommend that you talk to experienced skaters, study the magazine reviews, and then shop in a store where the staff are specialists in skates and fitting them. (If you can, rent skates to have some basis for decisions about features you like and don't like.) Make sure the boot will support your foot and ankle comfortably without constriction, and will wick out sweat. Selecting the wheels is tricky. Designs and materials vary according to use. No matter what you choose, make sure that you get a solid, smooth roll. The brake is critical. Don't leave the store before you understand how it works and have a good feel for the action.

Although in-line skating is an amazing cardiovascular cross-training sport and does good things for your lower body, we suggest that you supplement your workout with a good upper body program. Also, you would do well with some serious Active-Isolated Stretching work. Having a full range of motion in all joints and muscles in your body ensures that you can get into position (and, more important, get OUT of position) rapidly and completely. In-line skating is one sport that demands that you be in control, unless you want to be an aggro in a cast-o.

Skiing—Downhill

To Strengthen:	Upper Legs, Hips, and Trunk	1–15
	Shoulders	16–25
	Lower Legs, Ankles, and Feet	31–35

Coaches' Notes

Skiing is a big favorite of the Whartons because it combines aptitude and attitude with altitude. Nothing is better than a tuned athlete working out hard where the oxygen is thin. The body is forced to weave a few extra capillaries and generate a few extra corpuscles. If you've given all this inner activity enough time, you return to sea level literally supercharged with energy to spare for maximum performance. Besides, skiing is really fun.

Basically, the technique of skiing is to snap into your skis and poise with your feet slightly parted. Flex your knees, pressing your shins against the front of your boots, and lean slightly forward. This gives you the ability to use your hip flexors to transfer forces to your knees to absorb shock as you encounter bumps and depressions in the snow. Arms are in front of your body. Ski poles are in your hands. Point your skis down the mountain and you're outta here! Turning is a matter of shifting the weight off the back of your skis, cutting the edges into the snow, digging in, and creating an arc in the opposite direction. (The physics of turning are a lot easier to describe than they are to master.) Stopping is another matter altogether. (If we've made you think that stopping is really complicated, you're right. But we'll tell you a secret. It's the first thing that everyone conquers. No one wants to sail right past the warming hut on the first run and miss out on the hot chocolate!)

Assuming you already know how to ski (or just learned it all by reading the previous paragraph), we'll move on to physiology. Because skiing is a power sport that places great stress on the lower body, the most important muscle groups involved are hips and quads. The hip extensors, rotators, and flexors are the shock absorbers and the muscles that fire to weight, unweight, and direct the skis. The quads handle the load for powerful, strenuous, continuous action between the hips and those flexed knees. You use the lower legs for fine-tuning direction with pressure transmitted through your boots and bindings to the ski edges.

Downhill ski injuries are easy to study and track because nearly everyone who downhill skis does so in a resort, which has an emergency room and an orthopedic clinic right at the base of the hill. So our statistics and understanding are fairly comprehensive (as opposed to cross-country skiing, where the athlete can scoot out the back door and traverse a private area). Most injuries are of the lower leg, followed by the upper leg. Nearly a quarter of the injuries are likely to be fractures. Knees and ankles are highly vulnerable. And so are thumbs (from gripping the ski pole during impact).

A number of factors can reduce risk. The most obvious factor has to do with physical conditioning and training. If you're in shape and you're skiing at your level of ability, you dramatically reduce your risk. If you're not well conditioned and you leave your bunny-slope class to hit a black-diamond run (or ANY run that has the word "death" in its name), you're courting disaster. Make sure your equipment is in good shape, is appropriate for the type of skiing you intend to do, and fits you perfectly. Follow all the rules and adhere to all the safety codes of the resort, but ski defensively as if no one else will. Take note of the condition of the run. Well groomed and maintained snow is safer than a chopped-up course. And finally, try to quit for the day *before* you get tired. If you wait until you're pooped, your form will be sloppy, and you'll run the risk of someone skiing over your tongue.

We always advise our flatlander clients to be on the lookout for altitude sickness. At elevations between 8,000 and 11,000 feet, the weight of the air column above your head and the atmospheric pressure are less than at sea level. As you inhale, oxygen diffuses across the membranes of the air sacs (alveoli) in your lungs and into your blood. This happens because the pressure in the alveoli is greater than the pressure of the blood. This works well for flatlanders at sea level. However, at altitude, the pressure in the alveoli is less, and consequently less oxygen diffuses through the membrane into the blood. Your body could care less about your excuses. It needs and wants oxygen, so it takes matters into its own hands (so to speak) and starts adapting. You breathe faster and deeper, your heart rate increases, and your body transfers more blood to your brain (where you need constant and consistent oxygenation). Within five days, your body has produced extra red blood cells, myoglobin (intramuscular oxygen-carrying proteins in the red blood cells), and chemicals that help the oxygen combine with the blood cells. Within ten days, most people are pretty much acclimatized. Statistics show that the more fit you are, the faster you adapt. In the meantime, be on the lookout for warning signs of altitude sickness: unusual fatigue, drowsiness, weakness, headache, feeling faint, confusion, nausea, loss of appetite, accelerated heart rate, swollen hands and feet, tossing and turning instead of sleeping, and blue fingernails and lips. Rest, and drink plenty of water or sports drinks. If you develop a cough, get off the mountain and dial 911. Your lungs could be filling with fluid.

As fabulous as skiing is, it isn't a total fitness program. Also, even at its best, it's a seasonal sport. If you're going to be fit, you have to develop supplemental programs that you can use to juice up your skiing during the season and sustain your level of fitness during the off-season. You'll need broad adjustments during the year. You have to have a good strength program, with special emphasis on the upper body and the back of your legs. And you need to build a good Active-Isolated Stretch program to ensure a full range of motion for all your joints. You want to be as strong and agile as you can get.

Finally, a word about dehydration. It is deceptively easy to become dehydrated while skiing. Your body is losing water through exhalation and sweat, but you're hardly aware of it because you're in cold weather. And the telltale cotton mouth that serves as the first alert of dehydration is masked by the fact that your mouth is always dry when you breathe through it with exertion. This double whammy can mislead you. It's important that you drink before, during, and after skiing. Drink water or a sports beverage. An alcoholic hot toddy in the warming hut may warm your insides and quench your thirst, but it'll dehydrate you significantly, impede your reflexes, and cloud your judgment. Save it for later in the evening, at the lodge.

Snowboarding

To Strengthen:	Upper Legs, Hips, and Trunk	1–15
	Shoulders	16–25
	Lower Legs, Ankles, and Feet	31–35

Coaches' Notes

Snowboarding is the fastest growing winter sport in the world—and one of the fastest. (We're making this judgment based on the scorching speed at which snowboarders kamikaze past us skiers in the downhill!) Increasingly, mountains are the shared domain of both skiers and snowboarders because the requirements for lifts and runs are identical. And although the general idea in both sports is to get from the top of the run to the bottom, that's pretty much where the similarities end.

The equipment in snowboarding is a single "ski"—shorter and wider than either a traditional downhill or a cross-country ski. Ski poles are used only secretly in the first half hour of training. The skier mounts the board sideways, affixing both boots with bindings at various widths apart and at various angles, with the left boot forward. Variations in positioning are dictated by the type of boot (hard or soft) and the style of performance (from simple downhill to heart-stopping "extreme"). Every season brings new innovations in equipment and performance potential.

The physics of maneuvering a snowboard are an interesting cross between downhill skiing and surfing. The snowboarder controls acceleration and direction with subtle and not-so-subtle shifts in weight and foot pressure. These shifts originate in the hips and transmit all the way down through the knees to the feet. Equilibrium is maintained by flexing the knees and using the arms and upper body for counterbalance, much as a surfer does. Shock absorption is a function of hip flexors working in tandem with flexed knees to take the bumps and depressions in the snow. And all this takes place at breakneck speed.

Studies of snowboarding physiology and injury are relatively recent (as compared with other winter sports), but a couple of patterns have already become evident in the early stages of research. Most injuries present in inexperienced, young males under the age of twenty-one, and most injuries are on the left side. These statistical findings make perfect sense, because the sport, in fact, attracts young men who have to start somewhere. Unfortunately, we think they probably assume, "Hey! I ski, therefore I snowboard!" Dare we say it? Overconfidence has been known to cloud more than one young man's judgment. As for the injury rate being greater on the left side, this is easily explained by riding the board with the left foot forward. When a snowboarder falls, he or she either makes impact with the forward—left—side, or attempts to break the fall by thrusting the left arm and hand out. Sometimes, the arm breaks instead. But usually, the fall sprains or strains the wrist. Actually, fractures are number two on the injuries list. Most of the injuries occur in the lower body.

As orthopedists and sports medicine experts learn more about injuries associated with snowboarding, the industry develops safety equipment to protect rather specifically: wrist guards, knee pads, and helmets. Interestingly but not surprisingly, snowboarders tend to shy away from protective equipment. Consequently, we are continuing to see injuries that could have been avoided rather easily.

Although snowboarding is an exciting way for you to get pretty good cardiovascular and lower body workouts, it's not the perfect fitness program. The locked-down position of your feet does not allow the joints in your lower body to move in a full range of motion. In fact, the farther down your body you go, the more restricted is the movement. Hips are fair. Knees are poor. Ankles are bad. Feet are worse. Having your feet locked down forces you to fire your muscles in very specific, limited ways. For example, you might have killer quads, but your hamstrings will be weak and you'll have little development in your abductors and adductors—the muscles that move your legs to the outside or inside. Finally, your upper body will get no workout at all (except for lifting hot chocolate from the warming hut counter to your mouth). If you want to be truly fit, you'll have to supplement your program with flexibility and strength—all around. Also, extra cardiovascular work off the slopes will give you added stamina.

Soccer

To Strengthen:	Upper Legs, Hips, and Trunk	1–15
	Neck	26
	Lower Legs, Ankles, and Feet	31–35

Coaches' Notes

Every sport has its own peculiar perils. When an athlete from a specific sport calls for an appointment at our clinic, we have at our fingertips "The Wharton List" of potential injuries and physical difficulties that are likely to hobble through the door. Sometimes, we get surprised, but not often. The single exception to our ability to predict, and the one sport that keeps us from getting smug, is soccer. We NEVER have a clue before the athlete arrives, and we are ALWAYS surprised. Just when we think we've seen it all, here comes another oddball (uh, soccer ball) injury. Before you get the idea that we think soccer is out of control, be advised that we think soccer is a great sport that produces great athletes. In fact, it's the most popular sport in the world, played in nearly every country.

Soccer provides a wonderful cardiovascular workout that combines both aerobic and anaerobic activity. On the field, you're constantly on the move (this is aerobic). Even better, you frequently kick into warp drive (this is anaerobic). In fact, the workout provided by soccer is so intense that studies of top professional players reveal that they can completely deplete their glycogen stores during the course of a game. Glycogen is the energy fuel source your body stores and uses to fire muscles when the work is aerobic.

Not only are you getting a fantastic cardiovascular workout, but you're changing direction, accelerating, decelerating, and honing laser-sharp coordination and agility. The combination is a trainer's dream and a sports medicine physician's nightmare.

Because soccer is played all over the world and is enjoyed by men and women, children and adults, amateurs and professionals, it is difficult to generalize about the results of studies on soccer injuries. A few universal trends are evident, and none is surprising. Among all players, more than half of all injuries occur below the waist. Most injuries are bruises and sprains of ligaments and muscles. Ankles head the list. Goalkeepers are more frequently injured above the waist. Center forwards and midfielders are injured more frequently than anyone else. Older players get hurt more frequently and more severely than younger players. The more an athlete plays, the more likely he or she is to be injured. The higher the level of play, the more frequent and severe are the injuries.

Kicking—primarily instep kicking—can propel a ball at nearly 175 miles per hour. Biomechanical analyses of this famous signature kick have revealed that the force of the kick is sufficient to fracture a femur in midair, because the ball on impact absorbs only 15 percent of the kinetic energy generated by the leg, and the leg absorbs the rest—unless it hits the ground or another player, in which case all sorts of painful things are *certain* to happen.

Another way to advance the ball is to bounce it off one's head (or face). This is called "heading," and the average player will use this technique six times per game. All studies of head injuries related to soccer reach roughly the same conclusion—getting hit in the head with a soccer ball has consequences. Sometimes those consequences are immediate and painful. Sometimes they sneak up later, long after the player has hung up his or her cleats. For years, neurological researchers in the United States and Norway have been making some disturbing observations—that soccer players showed lower-than-normal average scores on tests for attention, concentration, memory, judgment, and overall mental functioning. Indeed, the researchers have been able to identify specific brain damage and atrophy directly related to the trauma of heading the ball. Not only is neuronal damage an issue, but physicians have been able to identify related chronic neck damage and significant decreases in the cervical range of motion. What might we conclude from all these studies? That repeated, high-velocity impact between one's head and a soccer ball isn't good. Protective helmets are not standard issue, so players should use caution.

You kick and head because you aren't allowed to use your arms and hands. The rule that you can't use the arms and hands, of course, is the single deficiency in regarding soccer as the perfect workout. If you're going to be totally fit, it is imperative that you include a strength program that gives attention to the upper body. Experts suggest that you use supplemental cardiovascular work to increase your endurance and train your body to conserve your glycogen stores. (We forgot to tell you earlier, when we cited that study of players who deplete their glycogen stores completely during a game—those players deplete gradually. As the stores drop, so does performance. A player who is sharp at the start is a mushroom at the end.) And no discussion about training for soccer would be complete without the strong suggestion that you practice Active-Isolated Stretching. The physical demands of this sport, combined with the need to change directions ballistically, mean that you need to have command of the widest range of motion you can get.

Finally, one of the greatest hazards of soccer—and the most easily remedied—is dehydration. Drinking a glucose polymer replacement fluid (one of the sports drinks) will help to keep you hydrated and to pump up glycogen stores, but it may be absorbed slowly into your system. And because the demands of soccer are going to put you into a heavy sweat right away, you can't afford the wait. You will do well to use the glucose polymer drink before and after the game, but rely on lots of plain, cold water during play. No matter what you choose, drink before, during, and after the game. If you feel thirsty, you're already well on your way to dehydration, so don't rely on cotton-mouth to signal you that you need to drink.

Squash

Coaches' Notes

One of our favorite client stories is that of a squash player who phoned us in a panic, announced that one of his arms was suddenly growing longer than the other, and made a hurried appointment to be evaluated before, as he said, "my knuckles drag on the court." When we sat down for our initial interview, we attempted to reassure him that imbalances between arms were not uncommon in racquet sports. Indeed, one arm gets a spectacular workout and the other one doesn't. This might make one arm appear longer than the other. Our new client interrupted our soothing theories. "Yeah, yeah, I understand all that. The problem is that the WRONG arm is getting longer." We glanced at each other, each hoping that the other Wharton had an appropriate response to such an insane remark . . . like there could POSSIBLY be a RIGHT arm to elongate. Jim was the first to break the stunned silence. He cleared his throat and plunged back in, "OK. Which arm should be elongating?" The client looked aghast, as if we were certainly the stupidest men in all of sports. "My racquet arm, of course. The centrifugal force generated by my swing combined with the weight of my racquet should be making that arm longer. But, that's not what's happening. The OTHER arm is getting longer!" He added wistfully, "If one of them has to elongate, it needs to be my racquet arm . . . ." Phil nearly choked, stifling the urge to break into hysterics. He couldn't resist leaning forward and asking confidentially, "What if what's happening is NOT that your nonracquet arm is getting longer, but that your racquet arm is getting . . . shorter?" That gave the guy something new and sinister to consider. Now the stunned silence was on the other side of the desk. We'll tell you right now that the story has a happy ending. Neither arm was shorter than the other. The client merely had muscle imbalances. One highly developed shoulder muscle group, a tight back, and a locked pelvis had drawn his racquet side up. The weaker side, underdeveloped, had stayed relaxed. When our client looked at himself in a full-length mirror and put his arms down at his sides, he could see that his fingertips on the racquet side brushed his thigh a little higher than his fingertips on the other side. The net effect was the illusion of elongation. The situation was easily remedied. Our client is balanced (both arms are equal in length) and we have a good story.

Squash gives you a spectacular cardiovascular workout, provided that you play hard and stay in constant motion. It helps develop eye–hand coordination, lightning reflexes, and the ability to stop, go, and pivot on a dime. It's an unparalleled stress buster because it burns up a lot of energy. It also gives you an opportunity for social interaction, always a plus in sports. And finally, it's relatively inexpensive, with low court fees and minimal equipment. We give it high marks for a sport of choice.

But, even though squash has high marks, it has some inherent risks. Rather than swinging the racquet (like tennis), squash players "slap" or "snap" it from the wrist. Because the racquet is lightweight, there is little impediment to this action. Consequently, we see a lot of elbow strain. In fact, the whole arm—from the shoulder to the hand—can be affected; tendons, ligaments, muscles, nerves, and bones are at serious risk. Most of these injuries are from overuse (the same damaging motion repeated frequently) or improper technique (swinging badly). And, if the player accidentally swats the wall with the racquet and stops the action midswing, the resulting trauma can be quite severe.

Injury prevention is a simple matter of being physically prepared to play. Remember that squash is a very fast game from the get-go, so warm up before you hit the court. Wear shoes that are specifically engineered to accommodate your pivot. Leave your running shoes in your bag. (Running shoes are disastrous for court sports. They're designed with a waffle pattern on the sole that helps keep a runner moving forward and backward—not side to side or in a pirouette.) Your shoes should be comfortable, yet snugly fitted. You don't want your foot to move within the shoe when you slam on your brakes and change direction ballistically. And you need good support to avoid shin splints and other related insults that plague the legs of squash players. Finally, wear eye protection to keep you safe from rocketing balls and flying players. Don't rely on your own glasses. You need the protection and comfort offered by the high tech eyeguards especially designed for racquet sports like squash. (In fact, most clubs and tournaments will require that you wear them.)

Although squash provides a great workout, it's not a complete one. Ask our client with the "long" arm! Any sport that places demand on only one side of the body has to be supplemented. You need strength work for the entire body, with a special emphasis on achieving muscular balance. This means extra upper-body work on your nonracquet side. Additionally, you will need Active-Isolated Stretching. If you play often (three times a week) and vigorously (you sweat for more than thirty minutes each time you play), you probably won't need an extra cardiovascular program. But, if you do put one into your workout, you'll be a much stronger player—guaranteed. If you don't play often or hard, you need to run, swim, or cycle.

Swimming

To Strengthen:	Upper Legs, Hips, and Trunk	1–15
	Shoulders	16–25
	Neck	26
	Arms, Elbows, Wrists, and Hands	27–30
	Lower Legs, Ankles, and Feet	31–35

Coaches' Notes

Maya Rogers came to us as a gifted runner who had a serious injury. In our judgment, she needed to lay off while we worked on it. But, like all runners, she was concerned that her training base would erode if she wasn't working out. And she was right. So we compromised. Maya would fully cooperate with a rehab program, and we would design an alternate workout regimen that would protect her years of investment. This was easy. We put her in the pool and carefully constructed a swimming program that maintained her fitness level without pounding her legs and hips. She did so well while she was with us here in New York that we had every reason to believe that she would do equally well on her own when she returned to Colorado. We phoned her a couple of months after she left our clinic and asked, "How's the running going?" Maya hesitated a moment and then said, "I'm not running anymore. I've quit." Our hearts stopped beating. These are words we NEVER want to hear. Quitting means failure. Total, complete, unequivocal, immutable failure. Both of us stammered, trying to find something to say that would be comforting and encouraging, something sensitive, gentle, and decidedly Wharton-like. It came out, "W-W-W-WHAT?!? Have you lost your freaking mind?!?" Then it was Maya's turn to placate. She laughed and said, "No. Swimming was a blast, and I'm pretty good at it. I've been invited to compete on a team here in Colorado, and practice takes all my time. I could run if I wanted to. I'd just rather SWIM!" We stopped hyperventilating, and performing the Heimlich maneuver and CPR on each other. Maya continued, "Thanks for turning me on to it!" So there you have it. Swimming is a blast.

There are four basic strokes in competitive swimming: the front crawl, the backstroke, the breaststroke, and the butterfly. The strokes have four common "phases": reach out, catch the water, pull the body using the resistance of the water, and recover by returning the body to neutral before beginning the phase cycle again. Although each stroke has its individual biomechanics, they all share one more thing in common: the shoulders, arms, and hands are under stress.

Shoulder injuries account for most of the injuries endemic to swimming. Little wonder. The shoulder is the most mobile joint in the body, and yet has little skeletal support. It relies instead on the shoulder capsule, the rotator cuff, tendons, ligaments, and muscles in the upper arm, shoulder, and upper back. It's an elegant relationship, but it breaks down now and then. Overuse injuries head the list with contributions from overtraining, poor training techniques, poor form in the water, fatigue, inflexibility, compromised blood supply to the shoulder, weakness, skeletal anomalies, untreated irritations and inflammations, imbalance, instability in the joint, and impingements caused by stroking. The possibilities seem endless and daunting, yet a little intelligence goes a long way in preventing injury.

Injury prevention begins out of the pool, with what swimmers call "dry land" training: strength, flexibility, and cardiovascular work. The next step is to work with a coach to be certain that your technique is perfect. Nothing will slow you down more or guarantee an injury faster than poor technique. Remember that perfect technique is hard on the body, but sloppy technique is dangerous. Next, be aware that overuse injuries can often be avoided by conditioning—working up to manage the demand slowly. Master one stroke before you move on to another. And be careful to gradually increase your time in the water. Fatigue is an important contributor to injury. If you're not physically ready to do the work, and you wear yourself out trying, you're headed toward injury. Finally, pay close attention to minor aches and pains, especially in the shoulders. Research demonstrates conclusively that shoulder problems start small. You might be able to head off a larger problem by dealing with a minor irritation.

As we said earlier, we often use swimming to keep endurance athletes like Maya fit while we rehabilitate injuries. Swimming provides a remarkable cardiovascular and muscular workout without pounding the joints. The support of the water takes all the weight off fragile body parts. This is why we also highly recommend it for formerly inactive older people who might not be well suited to hard charging. But this positive aspect of swimming is also a negative. Swimming is not "load bearing"; it doesn't give the bones the benefit of mild stress and gravity (such as would be found in walking, running, or cycling). Bones are living, dynamic tissues that regenerate and remodel themselves constantly. Those that are mildly stressed—loaded—rebuild more strongly and quickly than bones that aren't. The ability to help build skeletal integrity with exercise has significant consequences, especially later in life. For example, osteoporosis, the loss of calcium in bone, can be slowed and slightly reversed with load-bearing activity. Because swimming doesn't provide load bearing, you will find it necessary to engage in some dry land activities like walking.

Swimming isn't a perfect workout. Even elite swimmers put overall strength work into their programs, with a special emphasis on external shoulder rotators and upper back. Additionally, you will need Active-Isolated Stretching and supplemental cardiovascular work in your training regimen.

Finally, never let it be said, "Water, water everywhere and not a drop to drink!" Remember to put your full water bottle within easy reach and stay hydrated when you swim. It's easy to forget that you're working hard, heating up, and sweating while you're in cool water. But failing to maintain your fluids by drinking frequently will cause you to fatigue and lose function. We recommend drinking before, during, and after each workout. And, like Maya, have a blast!

Tennis

To Strengthen:	Upper Legs, Hips, and Trunk	1–15
	Shoulders	16–25
	Neck	26
	Arms, Elbows, Wrists, and Hands	27–30
	Lower Legs, Ankles, and Feet	31–35

Coaches' Notes

For two days, we played phone tag with Eric Thurmond. When we returned his phone calls, his housekeeper would always say, "Mr. Thurmond is in court. He has, of course, left strict orders not to disturb him unless there is an emergency. May I tell him you phoned again?" We assumed that he was either an attorney or a judge. When we finally connected with him, we were surprised to learn that he was, in fact, a music industry executive with a shoulder problem that was trashing his tennis game. Phil remarked, "Oh! We assumed you had something to do with the practice of law. You were in court every time we called." Eric laughed and corrected us, "I was ON the TENNIS court, not IN court. I guess it's obvious that I play a lot. My housekeeper tweaks the truth and protects my privacy by altering one small preposition. You're not annoyed, are you?" We totally understood. We work with athletes who are far sneakier and more creative than Eric Thurmond in carving out time for their sports. What did annoy us was that Eric was playing with an unevaluated shoulder problem. If he hadn't been on a serious losing streak, there was no telling how long he might have gone before he packed up his racquet—maybe for good.

Don't let the white outfits and genteel manners fool you. Tennis is one tough, blistering sport. During the serve, your shoulder internally rotates up to 1,715 degrees per second to give your racquet velocity up to 72 miles per hour. And a well served ball can rocket over the net at 125 miles per hour. Although your attention is generally drawn to the shoulder and arm, the swing actually originates with a ground reaction force in your legs that transmits up through your hips and back to your shoulders and arms. Your hips are the command center for that important rotation that winds the body up and then uncoils it to deliver power to a stroke. Your back bends and flexes in all directions—including obliquely—to facilitate the transmissions of power. Your legs create balance and bounce, running, stopping, changing direction, pivoting, and stabilizing. The demands on your whole body are enormous. And the workout is wonderful!

Understandably, injuries in tennis tend to cluster around the shoulder and back. Lower incidence of injury is reported in the elbow, knee, and ankle. Most injuries result from repetitive trauma—that is, getting pounded over and over until small insults accumulate and finally give way to injury. Accidents that result in such injuries as sprained ankles or broken bones are not uncommon. Some accidents are unavoidable, but to the extent that you do have control, you need to pay attention to small difficulties before they become big ones. A well-known coach once said, "Injuries are mistakes in your training." Don't make those mistakes.

Tennis is a great workout if you're a good player, and a great fitness program if you can play often. However, researchers record wide variations in expenditure of energy and workout benefit between recreational and elite players, between marginally fit and very fit players, and between singles and doubles players. So who you are and how you play will determine the extent to which you can rely on your tennis to deliver a fitness program. For the record, ALL tennis players are physically imbalanced, because of the overdevelopment of the racquet shoulder and arm. You need to compensate for that. At the very least, supplemental strength and Active-Isolated Stretching work need to be put into your program. If you want to improve your game, also insert a cardiovascular workout. Studies demonstrate conclusively that an aerobic program interspersed with short bursts of anaerobic work gives a tennis player an edge in maintaining stamina on the court. You want that edge.

Triathlons/Biathlons/Duathlons

To Strengthen:	Upper Legs, Hips, and Trunk	1–15
	Shoulders	16–25
	Neck	26
	Arms, Elbows, Wrists, and Hands	27–30
	Lower Legs, Ankles, and Feet	31–35

Coaches' Notes

One of our favorite riddles is: "Question: What's another term for 'injured runner'? Answer: Triathlete!" (If you're a runner, you too will think this is funny. If you're a triathlete, you'll think it's funny later.) Actually, the riddle speaks to the origin of the sport of triathloning. Endurance athletes fall into three main sports: running, swimming, and cycling. Historically, when an athlete was injured, he or she would switch from the sport of choice to one of the other two in order to maintain fitness levels. And switching within the three sports made a lot of sense, because each is radically different in terms of biomechanical demand. Runners, for example, could get off their legs, and swim. Swimmers could get vertical and take pressure off their shoulders, and cycle. Cyclists could uncurl and get off their fannies, and run. No matter where you worked within the three, you could get the spectacular cardiovascular workout that is the signature of an endurance sport. Over the years, athletes discovered great joy in the other sports, made considerable investments in new clothing and equipment, and developed proficiencies. Pretty soon, endurance athletes looked around and noticed that most of them could handle all three—running, swimming, and cycling. It was only a matter of time before these competitive athletes would design an event that combined them. Today, although distances and sportscapes may vary, the International Triathlon Union defines the standard triathlon as "an open water swim, a bicycle race on the roads, and a run on roads." In that order. Biathlons and duathlons are permutations of the triathlon, designating two of the three sports in various combinations. The great challenge of the triathlon is mastering all three sports. But the far greater challenge is being able to make successful, split-second transitions from one to the other.

For information on swimming, see page 175. For information on cycling, see page 118. For information on running, see page 155. For information on the transitions, stick around. It is said, "God is in the details." In the "athlon" sports, we think God is in the *transitions,* for as difficult and demanding as each individual sport is, making the instantaneous switch from one to the other is a killer. While you're

179

hopping through the parking lot, frantically ripping off your clothes and scrambling into a different outfit, your body is preparing to stage a major rebellion. It won't be pretty. And you'll deserve every painful minute of it.

Here's what happens. Most triathlons begin with the swim. Your body is horizontal and powered primarily from the shoulders, arms, and upper back. Your neck is flexed to get your face out of the drink. Your legs, although non-load-bearing, are generally straight and pumping from the hip flexors. If you've done well, you're likely operating at the anaerobic threshold. And although your core temperature is probably on the rise because you're working hard, you're relatively cool because you're wet. You're not drinking. You're pretty tired already. And metabolic waste products have begun to build in your body. Any "normal" person would rehydrate and rest here. But not you. Your job is only one-third done.

So you rocket out of the water, strip off your wet suit, run to your station, put on your cycling shoes and shorts, hop your bike, and speed off. Now your hands, arms, and shoulders are on the handle grips of your bike, supporting your weight. (Yes, these are the same fatigued hands, arms, and shoulders that, only seconds before, were powering your swim!) Legs that were extended and supported in water are now pumping pedals in a tight, tense cyclic pattern. Feet that were relaxed are now pressed onto hard pedals. Your back is hunched over the bike, supporting, stabilizing, and powering massive effort. You were hot in the water, but didn't know it. Now you do. Metabolic waste is building exponentially. When the ride is over, a "normal person" would—oh, never mind. You know what comes next.

You rocket off the bike, change shoes, smile for the camera, and then hit the road. Your back, fatigued from supporting, stabilizing, and powering cycling, is now getting pounded. Legs and feet that were pumping pedals and spinning are now propelling. They're hammered and shocked from the unforgiving, unrelenting, unyielding demands of the pavement. Arms and hands that were locked into position on the grips are now pumping to amplify the action of your legs. Lactic acid and metabolic waste from firing muscles build to levels that threaten to shut you down. Cramps threaten to turn you into a pretzel with one false move. Fatigue and pain cause you to question your sanity. Rational thought is replaced by one primitive, instinctive urge: Finish. And then it's over. You pick yourself up off the pavement to claim your trophy. IS THIS A GREAT SPORT OR WHAT???

In discussing injuries specific to each of the three sports, we direct your attention to the Coaches' Notes that deal with them. As we said, the variable that makes the "athlon" sports so interesting is the transition, and herein is the hotbed of injury—for good reason. Many athletes train for the sports specifically and individually. On Mondays, they swim. On Tuesdays, they cycle. On Wednesdays, they run. But stringing all three together in competition is radically different from training for one and then another. In fact, in "athlon" sports, the outcome is far greater than the sum of its parts. The body has to know how to change gears, switch muscle groups, and adjust to load. Successful triathletes train with a system known as "bricks." They put two of the three sports together in one workout, and shuffle the combinations. Like brick laying, you methodically place building blocks and cement them together until you have a strong completed project. "Bricking" works particularly well if you have limited time and a low "breakdown" threshold. Also, we advise you to train to balance your proficiency in all three sports. Try not to have either a strength or a weakness. Although it's difficult to resist having a "specialty," you'll do better if you're equally strong in all disciplines.

Remember to hydrate adequately. Also, because the triathlon can be an endurance event that places a high demand for energy, you might need to learn to take in some extra calories on the course. Many athletes use specially formulated food bars, bananas, and calorically enhanced sports drinks. Whatever you choose, be sure to practice before the competition, to make sure that you can handle the food and drink, and that your system can tolerate it. The last thing you want to add to your triathlon is "aerobic throwing up." Finally, remember that each sport individually is hard on your body. Stringing them together in training can easily cause overtraining. Be alert to signals such as weight loss, the sudden onset of colds, fatigue, moodiness, and a general ache that won't go away with a good night's sleep. The point is to have a good time!

Volleyball

To Strengthen:	Upper Legs, Hips, and Trunk	1–15
	Shoulders	16–25
	Arms, Elbows, Wrists, and Hands	27–30
	Lower Legs, Ankles, and Feet	31–35

Coaches' Notes

We had long been familiar with the name John Graham and already knew him to be a fine volleyball player when he called our clinic for an appointment to discuss difficulties he was having. We happened to be standing in the hall as he cautiously tiptoed toward the clinic door, so we both had the opportunity to observe his stiff, protected, tentative gait. He was obviously in a great deal of pain. Just to watch him made us both cringe. Once inside our office, he gingerly lowered himself into a chair, and we settled in behind the desk in front of him. We were feeling pretty smug and vaguely psychic, because we knew what he was going to say before he said it. We're trained professionals, after all. With years of formal education and field experience, we could merely observe him walk and KNOW (beyond doubt and without costly diagnostic procedures) that both of John Graham's adductors were injured—probably strained. Further, there was probably irritation of his gracilis, sartorius, and vastus medialis, which easily explained the stiff knees, the wide stance of the feet, and the difficulty in lowering his hips into the chair. And all this had happened in a single, violent moment during a volleyball game. We smiled benevolently and waited for him to confirm our insightful diagnoses. John Graham shifted painfully in his chair and said, "My right shoulder's locked." We both stiffened. Phil blurted out, "Your SHOULDER?!? What's with the tiptoe stuff and taking ten minutes to sit in a chair?!?" John grinned and replied, "Played in new trunks on the beach yesterday. Filled the liner with sand. Lots of it. You know . . . sand . . . trunks . . . ." He tilted his head toward his crotch and raised his eyebrows conspiratorially. We both recoiled. Not only were we instantly afflicted with "sympathy rash," but we were humbled. John Graham's britches had been filled with sand, and we were too big for ours. It just goes to show that there's a huge difference between the obvious and the apparent, especially when you're dealing with sports injuries and volleyball.

Without question, volleyball is a tough sport that places impressive demands on its players for explosive power, strength, flexibility, coordination, control, reflex, and stamina. Additionally, volleyball players are trained to focus completely and to make split-second decisions. The advanced training techniques deliver a stunning combination that develops some of the finest athletes in the world. Experts agree that, of all athletes, these tread a fine line: training to meet the rigorous demands of the sport, without overtraining and incurring overuse injuries. For this reason, professional coaches individualize the training programs and monitor them closely. There has to be team participation in skill development and play practice, but each athlete uses a tailored training program to protect his or her health and maximize individual performance. We advise you to use the professionals' approach to training. No matter what program you choose, remember that, in volleyball, there's no such thing as "one size fits all." Pay close attention to your own body so that you can train effectively without breaking down.

Injuries go with the territory. You can't dive through the gauntlet of elbows and knees to nail a ball spiked at 80 mph without endangering some vital body part. Contact and collision are par for the course. But the two leading injuries appear to be shoulder impingement (where the joint is traumatized, tissues swell, and function is shut down), and patellar tendinitis (the tendon at the knee cap is irritated or inflamed). Both are overuse injuries caused by repetitive action. The shoulder impingement is caused by hitting the ball. The patellar tendinitis is caused by jumping and landing. Because volleyball is a rough and tumble sport, and played without protective equipment, other areas of clustered, statistically significant injuries include feet, ankles, wrists, hands, fingers, hips, and lower back. To be honest, they are too numerous to list individually, but are collectively a warning that volleyball can be hazardous to your health.

Although we advise caution, we also encourage you to jump right in. Wear elbow and knee pads to protect yourself and others, and invest in a good pair of eye protection glasses. Volleyball is wonderful exercise and great fun. But like all team sports, it might take a bit of doing to get the gang together, so you might be limited to weekend participation. If this is the case, you need to do some supplemental training between matches. In fact, it's a good idea to supplement your game-day workouts, no matter how frequently you play. The pros do. You'll need sport-specific drills to develop the skills you'll need to win. And you'll need good strength, Active-Isolated Stretching, and cardiovascular programs. (Also, you need to practice shaking the sand out of your shorts, and if you see John Graham, remind him to do the same!)

Walking

| To Strengthen: | Upper Legs, Hips, and Trunk | 1–15 |
| | Lower Legs, Ankles, and Feet | 31–35 |

Coaches' Notes

It's hard for some professional trainers to take walking for exercise seriously. To be honest, we used to be among those people. It was a natural mistake. Walking isn't an Olympic event. It isn't even a sport. In fact, most of us regard it as basic transportation. But we Whartons have changed our minds. We've spent years studying it and documenting its effects on our clients. It took us a while, but we've seen the light. Today, if you ask us, we'll tell you that walking is one of the finest physical activities available to a person who is trying to get fit or to maintain fitness. Walking is a heart-pumping, head-clearing, muscle-firing, load-bearing, osteoporosis-quelling, joint-swinging, blood-circulating, lung-filling, artery-flushing, calorie-burning, fat-melting dream come true. It requires merely getting up out of the chair and moving forward. No equipment. No venue. No particular uniform. No special shoes. (In fact, you don't need ANY shoes. Bare feet will do nicely.) And you don't need coaching. (You got all the training you would ever need to be a champion walker by the time you were a toddler.) Pay attention now! It rarely gets better than this!

The mechanism of walking is simple. From a standing position, it's basically leaning forward from your ankles until falling on your face is a real possibility, and catching yourself before you do by sticking one foot out (heel down and toes up) to brake the fall. Then you transfer your weight to your front foot—the one you stuck out. And you lean forward again until you are once again in danger of falling. You thrust your rear foot forward to brake it. These acts of transferring weight from leg to leg and braking falls are steps. String a few of these together, and you've got walking. A really interesting dynamic of walking is arm-swinging as you stride. Left arm swings forward in synchrony with the right leg. Right arm swings forward in synchrony with the left leg. Swinging your arms (1) balances you as you shift your center of gravity from side to side and (2) amplifies the power in your legs in a fascinating, miraculous biomechanical relationship between two seemingly separate and unrelated functions. To see for yourself, try this. First walk with your arms straight down at your sides. Try to go faster without the assistance of amplification. Then, make it harder. Confuse your body by walking and swinging your right arm out with your right leg and your left arm with your left leg. (Good job if you can make it more than a few steps without losing your mind.) Finally, walk a few steps and notice the position of your arms—probably relaxed, and swinging only slightly. Then, walk faster for a few steps and notice that your arms naturally tighten up and swing in a more pronounced arc. Now, really power that walk and notice how your hands form fists, your elbows crook, your muscles tighten, and the arc of your arm swing is quite dramatic. Your body knows what to do.

Walking is mercifully easy on the body, but because it is, you may have to work hard to get your heart rate up in the "training zone"—that is, 60 to 80 percent of your maximum heart rate (approximately 220 beats per minute minus your age). While it's true that walking consumes the same number of calories per mile as running, you have to remember that it takes a lot longer to walk a mile than to run it. Running is, without question, more efficient in terms of time invested to get benefit. But that edge comes with a price. Running causes injury far more frequently and more severely than walking. Injured runners don't run. Injury-free walking rarely shuts down an athlete. You may not be fast, but you'll always be out there.

Now that we've applauded walking as a fabulous exercise, we have to admit that it's not perfect. You will need to supplement walking with a strength program—particularly for your upper body. And you'll need an Active-Isolated Stretch program to ensure that you have full range of motion in all joints.

We advise you to invest in the best shoes possible if you're going to make walking part of your daily routine. To turn walking from a good workout into a great one, warm up with stretching before you begin. Start slowly (for a few hundred yards at least) to give your muscles a chance to adjust to the work, and gradually build to the tempo you'll use throughout the walk. There are lots of ways to make the workout more effective. "Moseying" is useful, but gently increasing speed and distance will give you a better workout as your program progresses over time. In fact, once your body is used to one speed and one distance, it won't have to work as hard to get you there, and the benefits of the workout will deteriorate. Small periodic adjustments that make your workout just a bit harder will keep your body in a mode to work. And it's here, in this mode, that you receive all the benefit. When you're an experienced walker, try to include some hills in your workouts. A hill offers you an opportunity to use your muscles in a different way and puts an extra load on your cardiovascular system. If the hill seems daunting at first, and you console yourself by thinking, "What goes up must come down," you're right. But don't sell the downhill side short. It's as difficult as the uphill. Indeed, downhill walking makes surprising demands on the front of your legs and knees. If you can't find a hill, try walking up and down stairs. They work great. We don't recommend that you attempt to increase the difficulty of your workout by carrying hand weights or wearing Velcro wrist and ankle weights. Many studies have shown no benefit to walking with these weights. We feel that they place unnecessary stress on your heart by making you suddenly heavier at the same moment you're asking your heart to work hard. Also, they tend to upset the balance of your body and how you carry it.

Most important of all, walk safe. Like a pilot, "file a flight plan" before you walk. Tell someone exactly what route you're taking and when you plan to return. That way, if you don't show up, he or she will sound the alarm and know where to look. Also, vary your route and the times you walk, for your own safety. Predictable patterns make you vulnerable to crime. If you're walking at dusk or night, wear reflective gear. If you're walking on a road, keep to the left side, with traffic facing you. (Cyclists keep to the right side.) Drink cold water before, during, and after your walk, to avoid dehydration. Dress appropriately and comfortably, so that you neither freeze to death nor melt down. But mostly, have fun. We'll see you on the path!

Weight Lifting

Coaches' Notes

One of the first professional models we were hired to rehab was Inga, a shining Scandinavian woman with a million-dollar contract and an ankle the size of a grapefruit. She had to be carried into our clinic by her manager. The two of them were in a panic because Inga was scheduled to fly to Bermuda in two short weeks to shoot a choice bathing suit layout. Romping in the surf could probably be faked, and makeup could probably tone down the spreading bruise, but not even Inga's considerable charms in a bikini could distract the camera's lens from that swollen ankle. The opportunity of a lifetime was about to go down the drain in slow motion. Unless, hope beyond hope, we could fix it. We evaluated Inga and determined that, with patient work, we could get her to Bermuda with two ankles of equal size (small). We started to work immediately. Conversation naturally turned to the details of her accident. That morning, Inga had been posing for a book cover. The assignment called for a weight lifter to hoist Inga over his head, like a rigid human barbell. Both faced the camera. Everything was perfect in the lift. When the photographer was satisfied that he had the shot, he asked the weight lifter to gently lower Inga to the floor and stand her upright on her feet. Goliath's arms first trembled and then completely collapsed. He dropped Inga and she landed badly on one ankle. When Inga finished telling us the story, she asked, "How is it possible that he could lift me, but he couldn't let me down?" Our answer, "Very simply."

You only have to watch one competition on television to know that a weight lifter lifts the barbell, holds it for a set period of time (blink of an eye), and then steps back to let it drop to the floor. Inga's weight lifter had done what his muscles were trained to do. But Inga didn't do what a barbell does. She didn't bounce at his feet in a cloud of chalk dust. As opposed to body builders, weight lifters rely on strength and power to lift for one repetition at maximum weight. Olympic lifting has two lifts: the *snatch*, where the weight is lifted in a continuous pull from a position in front of the lifter's feet to above the head until the elbows are straight, and the *clean-and-jerk*, where the weight is pulled from the floor to the upper chest, stabilized while the lifter repositions his or her body to a standing posture, and then lifted over the head until the elbows are straight. The problem, of course, is that weight lifting trains an athlete to lift, but not to put down. These two biomechanical functions—lifting and lowering—use different muscles and different functions of the same muscles. The result of this specific training is a strong and powerful, yet imbalanced body.

Weight lifters should be in good shape before they engage in training. Lifting is hard on the body and can be dangerous. Competitive weight lifters have to watch out for elevated blood pressure, impaired cardiac function, headaches, fainting, varicose veins, phlebitis, hemorrhoids, bruises, scrapes, and calluses. In addition, lifters suffer from acute (traumatic) and overuse injuries that run the gamut. Trauma can often be prevented by being prepared, warming up before the lift, maintaining focus and concentration, working up to weight gradually, and practicing perfect form. Overuse injuries can be prevented with intelligently paced training, consistency, gradual building of weight and time, supplemental strength work to build the "unused" or "less used" muscles in the body, practicing perfect form, maintaining flexibility, and giving the body time to heal from injuries (large and small). To tell you the truth, we think the secret to success is a good coach who will help you maximize your performance and keep you from harm.

Weight lifting may give you strength and power, but it will also give you an imbalanced body. If you're going to be fit—TRULY fit—you need to round out your training with a supplemental strength program that balances your musculature, an Active-Isolated Stretch program, and a good cardiovascular program. Oh, and keep your hands off any human "weights" until you can pick them up AND put them down.

Wind Surfing

To Strengthen:	Upper Legs, Hips, and Trunk	1–15
	Shoulders	16–25
	Arms, Elbows, Wrists, and Hands	27–30
	Lower Legs, Ankles, and Feet	31–35

Coaches' Notes

A combination of surfing and sailing, wind surfing is a breathtaking hybrid sport that blends the best of the two into a spectacular experience. Speed, aerobatics, and turn-on-a-dime maneuverability are compelling attractions for athletes in search of challenge and excitement. Throw in a sunny day, a tubular wave, and a seagull or two, and you have perfection. It looks effortless. But looks can be deceiving. Wind surfing is, in fact, horrendously difficult.

As the wind shifts, wind surfing requires hair-trigger changes. You need midsection stability and upper-body strength and flexibility in order to pull and lift the sail into position. The front and back of your upper arms, shoulders, chest, and upper back are all under enormous strain as you counterbalance against the wind and the water. Your body has to stay erect and stable as you maneuver, so your trunk and hips serve as a sort of command center transferring power up and down your body, from your legs to your shoulders and back again as you shift. Your abdominals hold tight and keep you in position. You brace your feet on the board, with your toes gripping the surface, so that you have a firm base for your legs and hips. It's a tense balancing act that requires split-second timing and great agility. Like a gyroscope, you have to constantly find your "center" in fluid motion, and gauge the right amount of resistance and release to get your board to move. It's a fine partnership among the surfer, the board, the wind, and the water. When it all works well, it is poetry. When it doesn't, it's swimming.

We advise all wind surfers to be strong swimmers. Few things in life are as certain as this: you'll zig when you should have zagged, and end up in the drink. It happens to everyone. And, no matter how good a swimmer you are, wear a flotation vest, just in case the board comes down on your head.

Knocking your noggin notwithstanding, the injuries in wind surfing are few, probably due to the fact that when all hell breaks loose, you merely let go and fall into the water. Most injuries are related to strains in the upper back, shoulders, and upper arms, and most take place in one of two situations: sudden, unexpected wrenches of the sail, and straining to get the sail up out of the water when the surfer is recovering position on the board.

Another hazard of wind surfers is sunburn. When you're wet and rocketing through the surf with the wind in your face, it's easy to forget that it's hot out there and your skin is exposed to the sun. To avoid painful burns and the long-term risks associated with skin cancer, please use a waterproof sunscreen with the highest SPF you can find. (SPF 15 is the bare minimum.) Apply it in the morning before you step into the water, and reapply it frequently throughout the day, even if it's "waterproof." And remember that your eyes are exposed to the sun, too. Invest in a good pair of shatterproof sunglasses that filter out damaging rays.

Medical experts who track wind-surfing injuries note that wet skin is a problem. When your hands and feet are wet—particularly in salt water—they are depleted of their natural oils and become prune-like. The combination of oil depletion and shriveling makes the skin fragile. Gripping the beam with your hands, and bracing your feet on the surface of the board can cause serious irritations and abrasions. Be alert for tissue breaking down. Wear protective gloves and booties, and restore the oils with some high quality lotions at the end of your day.

Please remember to hydrate adequately. Again, it's easy to forget how hot it is out on the water when you're wet in the wind. Dehydration robs you of muscular control and causes fatigue to set in. You'll be more likely to make mistakes. Drink fresh water or a sports drink. And drink frequently. Avoid alcohol. It might LOOK like liquid and it might taste good on a hot beach, but it will dehydrate you. And worse than that, it will impair your judgment, coordination, and reflexes. You need to be 100 percent if you're challenging wind and water at high speeds.

If you're like a lot of wind surfers, you surf alone. We discourage this, pointing out that there is safety in numbers. Whether you're alone or with a buddy, before you go out on the water, tell someone where you're going and when you'll return. Wind is a fickle playmate. It has a wicked way of dying down and abandoning you when you need it most. You don't want to be stranded, alone, and without a fail-safe plan. It's nice to know that, if you're not in at a certain time, someone knows to come and get you. We suggest that you wear a waterproof watch (perhaps with a compass on it), along with your life vest, and adhere to your set schedule. It's also smart to wear some form of waterproof identification.

Wind surfing is a wonderful activity, but it's not a full fitness program. And it's probably reserved for your weekends, right? So, even at best, it's not a consistent workout. You'll need to do some supplemental strength to balance muscles that pull more than push and flex more than extend. And you'll need Active-Isolated Stretching work to get a full range of motion in muscles and joints that are fairly constricted. As for a cardiovascular workout, we suggest that you "kill two birds with one stone." Swimming should be a high-priority skill for you, so why not put together a swimming program that would hone your technique and build your stamina at the same time?

Wrestling

To Strengthen:	Upper Legs, Hips, and Trunk	1–15
	Shoulders	16–25
	Neck	26
	Arms, Elbows, Wrists, and Hands	27–30
	Lower Legs, Ankles, and Feet	31–35

Coaches' Notes

Darren Carson was a high school wrestler whose family contracted with us for a very specific goal: to bring Darren's wrestling performance to a championship level with an eye toward college scholarships. To be honest, because his parents had arranged for the program, we didn't expect the quality of commitment that Darren himself brought to the work. He trained with the single-minded focus of a man on a mission. The results were stunning. But he never warmed up to us. (Impossible to believe, right? We are, after all, Whartons.) Although we were together several times a week, Darren spoke only when spoken to. We thought he was merely a man of few words who was too focused to be bothered with the easy banter of a sports clinic and gym. Much later, we learned the true motivation behind his silent intensity. Darren wasn't working toward a championship, or to catch the attention of a scout, or to win a full scholarship to a major university. Darren was wrestling for vindication. Darren had been pinned on the mat by a girl. (Suffice it to say that it didn't happen a second time—but it could have if we had been training HER, too!)

Wrestling (in some form) is among the oldest competitive sports in the world, and it is part of the athletic heritage of every country on the planet. In western countries, we practice three primary forms: freestyle, Greco-Roman, and folkstyle. Although wrestling does have intricate and elegant elements, it's pretty basic: it makes a sport of primitive human fighting instincts that are as old as time. Interestingly, this "instinctive" origin presents a unique challenge to the training and rehab professionals who tend to forget that wrestling is combat, and wrestlers are combatants. Like all fighters, wrestlers are driven by inner voices that shout louder than any mere sports experts. We tell them to lay off, and they come on like gangbusters. We tell them to eat and drink to maintain life as we know it, and they starve and dehydrate to make weight. We tell them to rest an injury, and they give it five minutes before they're back at the edge of the mat. We tell them to wrestle by regulations designed for their personal safety, and they abandon decorum at the split second their opponents do. We ask them to tell us how they were injured and when, and they have no idea. These are not your usual athletes. These are wrestlers.

Statistics reveal that wrestling is second only to football in incidence of significant injury. Most injuries occur in practice (simply because wrestlers spend more time in practice than they do in matches), and most injuries occur when a wrestler is being taken down. Knees appear to be the most common sites of injury. No great surprise there. Because wrestling is a full contact sport (skin to skin), infections such as herpes simplex, impetigo, staph, and strep are easily spread. Hygiene—disinfected mats, fresh uniforms and equipment, and clean wrestlers—is important in preventing outbreaks.

Wrestling experts say that the most important ingredient in preventing injuries and infections is the coach. He or she is able to enforce adherence to rules and regulations, make sure that protective equipment is worn properly, and maintain hygiene. The value of your coach is then twofold: (1) to help you train to be the best wrestler you can be, and (2) to lay the groundwork to ensure your health and safety.

A note about making weight: A large percentage of young wrestlers do crazy things to lose weight before an important match. They believe they have good reason. Lightweight people wrestle lightweight people. Logically, there should be some real advantages to being a heavier person temporarily disguised as a lightweight. The takedown of that light opponent will surely be easier than wrestling someone equally heavy. So wrestlers cut their caloric intake to nil, exercise themselves into mush, sweat in saunas, suck down laxatives and diuretics, self-induce vomiting, shave their heads, cut their fingernails, and pick the threads out of their shorts. They'll drop those dreaded few pounds, but they'll also run the risk of cardiac function disturbances, heat stroke, and acutely impaired renal function. Not only is life on the line, performance is right alongside it. It takes up to forty-eight hours to replenish glycogen stores in the muscles, and twenty-four to thirty-six hours to recover from dehydration. Frankly, between the final weigh-in and the match, there isn't time to bring the body back to 100 percent. We join the American Medical Association and the American College of Sports Medicine in their condemnation of this practice. Our advice to you is to forget "making weight." Instead, be a great athlete so you can compete with peers. This is the only way you'll ever be sure how good you are.

Occupations

Driving

Coaches' Notes

In recent years, we've seen an increasing number of amateur and professional race car drivers in the clinic—not because they were injured and needed rehab, but because there is a growing realization within their profession that driving to win requires an athlete's stamina, strength, flexibility, physical control, coordination, and reflexes. But, unlike most athletes, drivers don't work in a field that has traditions for physical competitive standards and scientifically based training. Making the transition from "driver" to "athlete," however, is easy, because drivers well understand the principles for achieving maximum performance. Indeed, they've always applied them to their cars. They know that claiming the checkered flag is a matter of fine-tuning every variable under their control, down to the last bolt. Training the driver is much the same.

No matter what you drive, the fitness requirements—stamina, strength, flexibility, physical control, coordination, and reflexes—are the same. The problem is that driving gives you the ability to cover great distances without having to move at all. Too bad. The seats are engineered to cradle your torso and support your neck and head. Locked in. The seatbelt protects you from being thrown in impact, and restricts unsafe movement within the car. Locked in. Many of the car's controls are located right on the steering wheel and column, within reach without effort. Locked in. The console and dash are ergonomically designed to put all switches, buttons, and knobs at your fingertips. Locked in. You are able to roll down all windows and lock all doors with a flick. Locked in. Car phones are miked and voice-activated. Locked in. You can see what's beside and behind you by glancing at perfectly positioned mirrors. Locked in. The car's design is an efficiency engineer's dream come true—and a Wharton's nightmare. Although the car is designed to keep you locked into position, YOU were designed to move. When you're locked in, your body locks up.

The seat, no matter how plush and comfortable, puts enormous strain on your lower spine. Sitting is more stressful, in fact, than standing. Your back, hips, legs, and buttocks fatigue and tighten up. Once they tighten, they become even more fatigued. Other muscles engage to help compensate. Pretty soon, your whole body is entering into a vicious cycle of tighten-fatigue/tighten more-fatigue more, until muscles start shorting out and cramping. This is easily remedied by (need we say it?) MOVING once in a while. Take a break. Get out of the car, stretch, and walk a little to get your circulation going again. If it isn't practical to get out, at the very least shift positions in your seat to give your back a rest.

If you're going to be a good driver, you need to be a good athlete. Put together a fitness program that combines strength, flexibility, and cardiovascular work.

Keyboarding All Day

To Strengthen:	Upper Legs, Hips, and Trunk	1–15
	Shoulders	16–25
	Neck	26
	Arms, Elbows, Wrists, and Hands	27–30
	Lower Legs, Ankles, and Feet	31–35

Coaches' Notes

Our friend Bev is a medical writer in Florida, a devoted runner, and a rabid advocate for Active-Isolated stretching and strengthening. Last fall, we got an unusual phone call from her—at least we're pretty sure it was Bev. It was hard to tell because she was whispering. The conversation went like this: "Jim? Phil? You know who this is, but pretend like you don't. And if anybody asks, this conversation never happened, OK?" We solemnly agreed. She continued, "I need to know everything you know about carpal tunnel syndrome, but it's not me asking, right?" We were ecstatic. She was surely interviewing us for some article she was ghostwriting for a high-profile client. We asked, "Are you writing another piece on carpal tunnel syndrome? Why are you asking US about it? You write about it all the time. In fact, we consider you to be the world's leading lay expert. Do you just need quotes or something?" She whispered hoarsely, "Uh, yeah. I need quotes. Let's say there was this . . . uh . . . writer whose hands were curled into claws and she was paralyzed from the elbows down and . . . ." Her phone clattered to the floor. We listened intently as she clumsily retrieved it and apologized. We're not stupid. We suddenly realized that our friend was asking about herself. Never ones to let a delectable moment slide by, we set the trap. "Bev, did you develop carpal tunnel syndrome WHILE you were writing a piece on carpal tunnel syndrome?!?" Indignantly, she snapped, "No, of course not!" But we know her too well. We circled for the kill. "Now, Bev, come on. You can tell us." She caved. Her strangled reply was, "I was writing a piece on carpal tunnel syndrome PREVENTION." We had to call her back. We were laughing too hard to be of any use to her. Besides, we had to savor the moment.

Carpal tunnel syndrome is a "cumulative trauma disorder" or a "repetitive stress injury," meaning that a small, seemingly insignificant trauma delivered over and over accumulates until it causes a problem. These injuries aren't limited to computer keyboarders like Bev. It's been called the "Workplace Epidemic." In fact, as early as 1989, OSHA declared that virtually EVERY workplace in the United States had potential for repetitive stress injuries. Today, more than half of all work-related, reported "illnesses" are repetitive stress injuries, creating an enormous drain on workers' compensation dollars. It's a potential problem for *anyone* who does repetitive tasks—cashiers, musicians, assembly line workers, and so on. (We even treated one guy who got carpal tunnel syndrome from using his channel changer!)

Prepare yourself. We're going to tell you something shocking that Bev already knew. If you have carpal tunnel syndrome, it's your own fault. You caused it. Wait! Before you mail us your wrist braces inscribed with death threats, let us explain. Carpal tunnel syndrome is a classic overuse injury—and it's easily preventable. People aren't suddenly struck down without warning. Indeed, it happens slowly, over a long period of time, while a person ignores clear signals that the body sends to alert its owner that "things aren't right." The first signal is fatigue. The response is simple: take a short break every hour to improve circulation, change position, and restore range of motion. Also, it helps if the keyboarder, like any athlete, is physically fit with specific training to withstand the demands of the job. Keyboarding requires strong arms, shoulders, and back, and flexible wrists, hands, and fingers.

Carpal tunnel syndrome isn't the only culprit waiting to disable a keyboarder. Just when you thought it was safe to go back to the keyboard, we've got yet another problem to discuss. People who operate keyboards are seated and stationary for long periods of time. Sitting in a chair—no matter how high-tech and perfectly fitted it is—places enormous strain on the body from the neck down the spine through the shoulders and hips. Immobility tends first to fatigue muscles and then to lock them up. That signature fatigue and tension between the shoulder blades of keyboard operators are classic examples of the consequences of sitting in one position without moving. Trust us when we tell you that it just gets worse as it spreads.

When you spend all day keyboarding, you aren't getting enough exercise. You must develop a total program that includes strength, Active-Isolated Stretching, and cardiovascular work. Finally, when you're on a keyboard, MOVE once in a while. (And if you see Bev, ask her about her claw-paralysis thing, but don't tell her you heard it from us.)

Lifting and Hauling All Day

To Strengthen:	Upper Legs, Hips, and Trunk	1–15
	Shoulders	16–25
	Neck	26
	Arms, Elbows, Wrists, and Hands	27–30
	Lower Legs, Ankles, and Feet	31–35

Coaches' Notes

One evening, while we were working at a sports expo here in New York, we met a young man who expressed more than casual disdain for the fervent zeal of the exhibitors and sports enthusiasts who cruised the booths, collecting materials and samples. He had been dragged along by friends. As he postured and snarled about "rip-offs" and "wasting time," we listened politely (and suppressed the urge to gag him with a sweat sock). We hate it when someone's ignorance entraps him in an unhealthy body. We thought we might break down his resistance with a little charm and a demonstration of how easy and enjoyable it can be to get fit, so we invited him into our area for a courtesy workout. He said, "No thanks. I work at a warehouse all day, lifting and hauling. And I do fine. I don't need all this hype and expensive junk. I wear this." He opened his jacket to reveal a wide, black, neoprene "back support" belt that fastened around his (rather large) waist and was held in place by suspenders. He pirouetted so that we could admire it from all sides. Across the back was stenciled "Safety First!" in large yellow letters. We smiled politely and handed him our card. He closed his jacket with a snap, sneered at us, stuffed the card into his bag, and lumbered off. We didn't give him another thought. Until about two months later. He sheepishly phoned us. Seemed that he had thrown his back out. (No!!! What a shock!) The company doctor had ordered him to rehab—and delivered a further mandate to get in shape or else! He wondered if we could forgive him, and take him on as a client. You bet we could. And did.

When we define "fitness," we say that it is comprised of four components: health, strength, endurance, and flexibility. If you are to be truly fit, you have to have all four components in place. One might outshine another, but, to some extent and in some balance, all four are linked and important. When, like our belted young man, a person relies on one to the detriment of the others, then problems set in . . . particularly if the person is engaged in physically demanding activity like lifting and hauling. And worse, because the person "works" all day, he or she might be deceived into thinking that this is a "fit" body. Wrong. It's possible to work hard (for a short career) and look great, and yet be unfit. It's only a matter of time before something gives.

Lifting and hauling place specific stress on specific muscles within the body. Those muscles that are being used get strong, and those that aren't, don't. The result is muscular imbalance. The problem is that most lifting and hauling takes place in the front of the body, with the lower back and hips assisting. The back, buttocks, and hamstrings stay in contraction to support effort until fatigue sets in and muscles start shorting out. When those muscles can no longer do their jobs adequately, muscles in the front of the body work harder to take up the slack. But they'll quickly fatigue with the ever-increasing load. Imbalance is a problem not only from muscle to muscle, but also within individual muscles. Lifting, for example, gives your shoulders and arm muscles good workouts as you lift UP. Putting something DOWN is an entirely different story. The muscles you're using have developed only half their functional strength. They can flex (lift) effectively, but they can't extend (lower) as strongly. When muscles go into failure, the body scans for other muscles that can be recruited to compensate, and the person will make decisions to change the way he or she moves to get the job done with new and less effective postures and techniques. It's like a ticking time bomb, a countdown to disaster.

Injuries in lifting and hauling can be both traumatic (like strains and sprains) and related to overuse (like tendinitis). The statistics generated by sports medicine experts who evaluate the biomechanics of lifting and hauling indicate that injury sites and possibilities are unremarkable. We find exactly what we expect: lower back, shoulders, biceps, deltoids, elbows, forearms, wrists, hands, groin, quads, hamstrings, and buttocks. While you were taking personal inventory, did you notice the one interesting exception? Lower legs. Knees, ankles, and feet don't appear to be in as much jeopardy as upper-body soft tissues such as back, shoulders, and arms. It is possible to injure a knee, ankle, or foot, but doing so requires bizarre circumstances, creativity, and a radical mistake.

Don't lift or haul until you are physically ready for the challenge, and fully fit. And we're going to tell you what we told our belted young friend: "Lose the belt." Many insurance and sports medicine statistics don't support the belt manufacturers' claim that using a belt will prevent back strain. On the contrary, relying too heavily on a belt deceives you into thinking that you're protected (so you try to do more than your body can support), alters your biomechanics, and keeps you from doing the work you need to do to get those muscles strong. In defense of belts, they will keep your waistline warm in a cold warehouse, and they will remind you to maintain good posture. Buy a sweater and listen to your mother. Take the belt off. If you have to wear something, we suggest gloves to protect your hands.

Get thee to the gym! You have to develop a fit body if you're to do your job well and without injury. As we said earlier, lifting and hauling tend to build an unbalanced body, and you don't want to be regarded as *unbalanced*. Also, put an Active-Isolated Stretching program into your routine so that your muscles and joints can have the benefits of a full range of motion. Not only are flexible muscles easier and quicker to move, but they'll help you sidestep a falling crate. And finally, lifting and hauling are not aerobic. You should put a good cardiovascular workout into your fitness regimen. Try brisk walking, running, cycling, or swimming for thirty minutes, at least three times a week.

Pushing and Pulling All Day

To Strengthen:	Upper Legs, Hips, and Trunk	1–15
	Shoulders	16–25
	Neck	26
	Arms, Elbows, Wrists, and Hands	27–30
	Lower Legs, Ankles, and Feet	31–35

Coaches' Notes

We train all sorts of athletes, but we had never been approached for a maximum performance fitness program tailored to handle "rough mating" until we got a call from Kirk. To be honest, we weren't really interested in evaluating the biomechanics of his kinky practices and then helping him prepare. We were going to thank him for his interest, but suggest that he contact someone else. When Kirk came in for his intake interview, we could scarcely reconcile his demeanor with his bizarre request. Before us sat a soft-spoken, apparently mild-mannered gentleman. Indeed, his registration form stated that was a professor at a major university. We exchanged pleasantries with the intention of leading the interview to a very rapid conclusion, when Kirk stopped us dead in our tracks by flatly stating, "I don't need to tell you fellas, it can get pretty rough." He had a faraway look in his eye, and shook his head slowly. Being "guys," we shuffled our feet and shifted in our chairs in silent commiseration. He continued, "It's all huffing and pawing and straining at the ropes." We froze in mid-shuffle and shift. Kirk took no notice, and continued, "In the heat of passion, blind instinct just takes over. Why, one time last week, it got so wild that I got jerked off the wall and stomped." He lifted one sandaled foot for our inspection. "Broke my toe. Hey, I'm not worried so much about me as I am about one of them getting hurt." *(There was more than one?!?)* Kirk said, "They cost up to a million dollars each." *(These were some high-priced lovers!!!)* We knew we couldn't let him continue, no matter how intrigued we were. Jim interrupted, "Kirk, we understand your difficulties, but we really don't think we can participate in something as 'personal' as this." Kirk stared at us in disbelief, "This isn't personal, gentlemen. It's professional." Jim said, "Even more reason for us not to be involved. I'm sure you can appreciate our need to protect the reputation of our practice, so if you'll excuse us . . . ." We both stood up. Kirk burst out laughing and choked, "I'm a professor of equine veterinary medicine. I'm a *horse* doc! I specialize in genetic engineering. I'm talking about collecting sperm, and mating championship stallions and mares all over the world!" There was nothing we could say that would excuse the fact that we might have known all this if we had read past line 2 on his registration form. We waited until our new client had finished rolling on the floor and guffawing, and then we three embarked on a fitness adventure that would take us from the clinic to the plush stalls of a university genetic engineering facility.

Handling horses in (and out) of the throes of passion requires great strength and control. Kirk needs to guide them into very restricted specialized stalls, to station them exactly, to correct and adjust if they shift out of position, and to be able to react to protect himself and his assistants against sudden, unexpected movement. Kirk is a classic example of an occupational athlete. His job requires him to develop overall fitness with emphasis on pushing and pulling. Helping a horse move forward required pulling. Helping a horse move sideways or backward required pushing. And Kirk needs to be strong, balanced, and flexible, and have plenty of stamina to handle the physical demands of a long day in the barn. It was a tall order for a vet who never expected to see the inside of a gym, but certainly possible—and entirely necessary to prevent any more bone-shattering stompings. We've heard that "love hurts," but this was ridiculous.

There are a few rules for men and women who, like Kirk, work in professions where pushing and pulling are required. You have a professional responsibility to be fit to do your job. First, get in shape and maintain that fitness level with a regular program. Anything less than this, and you are liable for putting yourself and others at risk of injury. Second, get a handle on the physics of your tasks. Thoroughly understanding what kind of force, and how much it will take to move an object, will give you ideas about the best ways to use your body. Third, get advice from more experienced professionals who have had more time to work out shortcuts and tricks. And finally, take smart advantage of tools, equipment, and protective clothing. It's stupid to insist on being a purist if there's help available.

Pushing and pulling fire the front and back of your upper arms, chest, and upper back. While you're positioning your body, your trunk muscles hold you erect, stabilize your posture for leverage, and assist movement such as bending, twisting, and reaching. Your abdominal muscles help you bend forward, and your lower back helps you flex backward. Because pushing and pulling are largely about leverage, you have to stabilize yourself, using the stance of your body or an immovable object—such as a wall or a fence rail—to counterbalance the force of your movement. Even though the power seems to be centered in your upper arms and chest, your whole body gets involved—through your hips and legs, right down to your toes.

In spite of the total body involvement, this isn't a total workout. Pushing and pulling, no matter how long and hard, aren't going to help you build a balanced, fit body. The action is too specific and biomechanically restrictive. You'll need supplemental strength work to give all your muscles a chance to fire. Additionally, you'll need Active-Isolated Stretching to give you a full range of motion for rapid, controlled action (like getting out of the way of a horse's hoof). And finally, you need to increase your stamina by rounding off your program with a good cardiovascular activity such as running, walking, swimming, or cycling. Although you're getting into shape for your work, you'll find that it will be lots of fun. Think of it as "horseplay"!

Sitting All Day

To Strengthen:	Upper Legs, Hips, and Trunk	1–15
	Shoulders	16–25
	Neck	26
	Arms, Elbows, Wrists, and Hands	27–30
	Lower Legs, Ankles, and Feet	31–35

Coaches' Notes

For a while, we were getting an unusual influx of "weekend warriors" into the clinic. Executives, clerks, and secretaries formed a seemingly endless procession of poor souls who had gone out to play on the weekend and had ripped, torn, spindled, or mutilated some body part vital to life as they knew it. The clinic staff could hardly keep up with the demand. We would no sooner shore up one "weekend warrior" when three more would hobble in. When we remarked to a friend that this seemed to be a losing battle, she told us the story of a physician who was walking beside a river and noticed a person struggling in the current, yelling for help. The physician jumped in and saved the person from drowning. When the person was safely on shore, the physician continued his walk beside the river. Minutes later, a second person swept past him in the water, struggling and yelling for help. A second time, the physician dived in and rescued the person from drowning. When the second person was safely on shore, the physician continued his walk. Minutes later, a third person called to him from the currents. When he had finished this third rescue, the physician thought, "I can't continue to jump into the water to save drowning people. I need to run upstream and stop the guy who's throwing these people into the river." In other words, he needed to tackle the problem at its source and fix it, rather than resign himself to endless rescues. The point was clear to us. We needed to *prevent* the injuries. So, we intensified our efforts in basic training and conditioning, making the work specifically available and accessible to men and women employed in offices. It didn't take long before we got the results we needed.

The purpose of fitness is much more than preventing injuries. But, for people who sit all day, prevention is a critical benefit. Sitting all day is a crime of both commission and omission. It's terribly hard on your body, and yet, as long as you're sitting, you're not working your body. Frankly, it's our own fault. We've created this irony by insisting on efficiency. Industrial efficiency experts and ergonomic engineers have designed easy-to-use workstations that place everything within reach. Electric staplers and pencil sharpeners. Drawers that glide with the tap of a finger. Voice-activated electronics. Lights on automatic switches. Feather-touch computer keyboards. The evolution of efficient space and equipment is wonderful, but using them has sinister consequences. With every energy-saving trick we pull, we lose one more opportunity to use the body as it was intended, and we move one step closer to profound injury. At some point, we'll surely hit the law of diminishing returns. Good thing we've saved all that time and energy! We'll need it for rehab to restore tone and control to bodies that have deteriorated into oatmeal.

And it's not just all the things we DON'T do that are causing us problems. The way we use the body contributes to injury. Working on a desktop directs effort and attention directly down in front of the person, at just above waist level. Studies have shown that desk dwellers rarely organize their work to expand beyond that riveting eighteen-square-inch area. Assuming that the task is interesting, the worker probably will move very little during the course of the shift. Hands and lower arms are up on the desk, which places strain on the upper back and shoulders. The neck flexes forward and likely locks into position for long periods of time, further fatiguing the upper back. The abdominals relax. The spine flexes as the person leans forward toward the desktop. The chest compresses slightly, and breathing becomes more shallow. Sitting in a chair—no matter how well designed and perfectly fitted it is—strains the lower back. (In fact, sitting is harder on the body than standing.) The net effect of these small physical compensations is one huge problem.

Sitting at a desk all day does nothing to build you into a vital, healthy person. Years ago, an executive from a leading corporation consulted the Fatigue Laboratory at Harvard. He complained that his management team was losing out in bargaining with labor on the basis of "sheer physical force," and he was looking for a solution. He said that bargaining was a marathon. His management executives smoked and drank, and didn't exercise or get enough sleep. On the other side of the bargaining table were the blue-collar workers, who were in better shape and healthier. Invariably, at the end of a very long day of stressful negotiating, the management executives would slide into comas at the same time the blue-collar guys were just getting warmed up. Both sides knew this was going to happen in advance. No matter how well armed management was, at the end of the negotiation session, the blue-collar guys would rev up and pound the table, and the management team would cave in from sheer exhaustion. They would agree to anything, just to get out of the conference room. The executive who came to Harvard for a solution was tired of being physically overpowered in business meetings that had nothing whatsoever to do with physical capability. He was wrong about fitness and business, but he was right about recognizing the power of strength and stamina.

Our advice to people who sit all day is to knock it off. Use every excuse you can think of to get up and move once in a while. If your supervisor frowns on jogging around the desk, at the very least, shrug and roll your shoulders hourly. Stand up and stretch to take some of the pressure off your hips. Take a deep breath. Straighten out your knees and wiggle your feet to get circulation moving again. And dial your touch-tone phone to make an appointment with the nearest fitness center. You have work to do. You need a strengthening program, an Active-Isolated Stretching program, and a good cardiovascular program. Now.

Standing All Day

Coaches' Notes

We were once contacted by a sports medicine physician who asked us to take one of his patients into rehab on an emergency basis. Before we agreed, we needed a little more information and inquired, "Her problem?" The physician corrected us. "Problem*s*." He said, "She has severely strained plantar fascia in the arches of both feet, a calcification at the point of strain on her right heel, and related pain in her knees, hips, and back." We were impressed. These kinds of snowballing injuries occur when an athlete is really pounding. We asked, "Is your patient a competitive marathon runner? A professional soccer player? A dancer?" The physician replied, "Checkout clerk at a grocery store." Now, we were REALLY impressed. We had no idea that checking out groceries could be such an occupational hazard, but we were soon to get an education on the severe consequences of combining a concrete floor with an eight-hour shift.

The human foot is a remarkable shock absorber. When you put weight on it, it literally converts the vertical force of your weight to longitudinal force by distributing it throughout your foot. Your arch is like a spring. As you walk, you put weight on your foot and compress the plantar fascia—a long elastic cord on the inside of your foot—between the ball of your foot and the front of your heel. It flattens slightly to absorb the shock of your step and make your landing "spongy and soft." When it's stretched to its full length, it's tense, ready to put "spring" into your step to help you push off. As you move forward through your stride and take the weight off that foot, the arch does indeed return to its neutral position. When you stand for long periods of time with the arch in full extension—flattened out—the muscles around it fatigue. They're expecting you to move. When you don't, they are overworked and strained. When they short out, your body will recruit other muscles to take up the slack. When those fatigue and short out, other muscles try to compensate. You get the "snowball" effect: injury begets injury. Eventually, the compensations will spread to the hips and back, as they did with the grocery store clerk.

Another problem with standing for long periods of time is that your circulation becomes "sluggish." Fluids accumulate in lower extremities, and metabolic waste from fatigued muscles cannot be flushed properly.

The accumulation of fluids causes swelling, and swelling causes discomfort. The final insult is that gravity and inactivity can exact a serious toll. If blood doesn't get to your head in sufficient supply, you can become faint. (Remember the guards at Buckingham Palace, who are famous for standing at rigid and royal attention—and then keeling over on their faces?)

We recommend good footwear. Whether you are wearing shoes or boots, they need to fit properly and provide support that is appropriate for the surface on which you work. If you're in doubt, ask advice and take careful notes from the coworker who looks the most comfortable and leaves the workstation at the end of the shift WITHOUT limping or grunting.

Standing all day will not give you a good workout, so you will need to put together a comprehensive fitness program that provides strength, Active-Isolated Stretching, and a good cardiovascular workout. Also, during the course of every shift, move. Walk in place, wiggle your toes, or shift your weight from one foot to the other, resting a tired arch.

Part IV

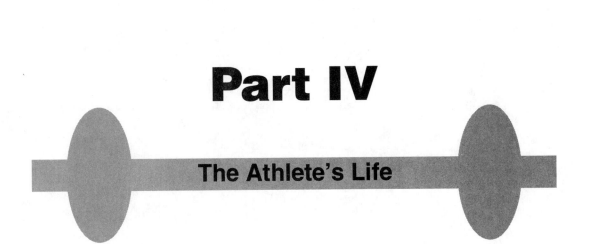

The Athlete's Life

Eating Like an Athlete

One of the greatest rewards of working out and burning calories is that you now have permission to EAT! In fact, we insist that you dig in! Want to get REALLY excited? Endurance athletes, such as competitive marathon runners, consume up to 6,000 calories a day and stay lean. But before you skip out and load your freezer with ice cream, we have to have a serious discussion about responsibility. As you become fit, a subtle change starts taking place in your relationship with all food. When you become more attuned to your body and its ability to perform, you'll start noticing that you're naturally gravitating toward food that's good for you. You'll shift from looking at food as "entertainment" and start regarding it as "fuel." You'll select things that provide calories and nutrients rather than crunch and comfort. Some of our clients say that this evolution starts with guilt. After they've put in time on their workouts and experienced the exquisite satisfaction of results, they have a moment of truth—usually while shouting into the clown's mouth at the drive-up window of the local hamburger joint. Suddenly, it occurs to them that they're trashing all their efforts by loading up on junk. And they're doing nothing to fuel their bodies for the next workout. Then, because they're tuning in to their bodies, they begin to notice a "craving"—an undeniable attraction—for *broccoli* and other formerly nauseating things. Don't laugh! It'll happen to you, too. But before you curl into the fetal position around your beloved cupcakes, be advised that a successful eating plan for an athlete includes an occasional "slip" into former, wicked ways. One famous marathon runner is quoted as saying, "Without ice cream, there is darkness and chaos." We couldn't agree more. So, before we begin this lesson in how to eat as an athlete, we're telling you in advance that you are permitted to dive face-first into junk food *once in a while.* Athletes are NEVER on diets. They're eating intelligently.

Professional athletes eat at a "training table." This means that, when they sit down to eat, the food in front of them is an integral part of their commitment to their athletic program. Balance is the key to healthy eating throughout your life: eating a balanced diet, and balancing your nutritional requirements against your calorie and fat intake. As mounting evidence by researchers links diet to disease prevention and treatment, you can be certain that what you eat has a direct effect on your health. A good diet reduces the risk of premature death from our biggest killers: heart disease; high blood pressure; some cancers such as endometrial, breast, and colon; stroke; and non-insulin-dependent diabetes. In addition, there are some real benefits to getting your weight under control. Lowering body fat decreases the risk for diseases linked to obesity, makes it easier to recover from surgery, and, later in life, helps deal with complications from arthritis, and helps keep a person mobile and on balance.

It's up to you. There is no better time to get started on a healthy diet. It's never too late to make important improvements, and you want to take control as soon as possible because there is evidence that the pounds you put on in your middle and later years are more hazardous to your health than extra weight you've carried since childhood. Studies have demonstrated that people who gain weight in their middle and later years are more likely to develop heart disease—the country's number one killer—than people who have been overweight since childhood. Additional research suggests that the statistical increase in heart disease in older women may be linked not only to the natural decline in estrogen (which has cardioprotective effects), but also to carrying excess weight—no matter when you put it on. An eight-year study of 115,886 women 30 to 55 years old has clearly demonstrated that coronary events such as fatal and nonfatal heart attacks were linked to being overweight.

GET YOUR WEIGHT UNDER CONTROL DURING YOUR MIDDLE YEARS

"Middle age spread" is one of the very real challenges of older people. It is called "creeping obesity" because it happens slowly, due to metabolic changes that occur naturally during aging. By the time you're age thirty, your metabolic rate (the rate at which you burn calories) starts to decrease by about two percent per decade. By age eighty, you're burning 200 fewer calories than you did when you were thirty. Simple math would suggest that merely eating 200 fewer calories per day should keep weight level, but it's not that simple. Most people also tend to decrease their activity levels, so the energy demands made by their bodies are diminished. Decreased activity also causes muscle mass to decline. Muscles are the big calorie-burners in your body, and when muscle mass declines, your need for calories diminishes. The net effect is weight gain. The heavier you get, the less you tend to move. The less you move, the more weight you gain. It's a vicious cycle.

SO YOU'VE TRIED DIETING ALL YOUR LIFE AND FAILED?

The other vicious cycle in personal weight management is crash ("yo-yo") dieting: gaining and losing, gaining and losing. When you drop your calorie intake quickly or dramatically, your body is programmed to translate your new diet as "All systems alert! We're starving to death!" and undergoes a series of adaptive changes—literally slowing down systems—to conserve energy and calories. Your body, wonderfully efficient and adaptive, gets better and better at dropping into its "conservation mode" every time you go on a low-calorie diet. Even if you do manage to lose weight, when you go off your diet and return to "normal eating," you gain weight back quickly and may gain back more than you lost. Your body has slowed down a little to conserve energy, and it requires still fewer calories than when you started. That's also why it's harder every time to lose weight. As discouraging as this is, the National Institutes of Health has some good news for you. Most studies have shown that weight cycling does not affect your long-term metabolic rate (the rate at which you burn calories). More important, the fact that you've cycled will not adversely affect the success of your future diet attempts. Additionally, weight cycling neither increases the amount of fat tissue in people who lose and regain weight, nor does it add abdominal fat. No matter how many times you have failed in the past, a new attempt just might be the one that succeeds.

HOW MUCH SHOULD YOU WEIGH?

There are general guidelines, but everyone is a little different and the ranges can vary from person to person. How much you weigh seems to be less important than your total body composition and how much fat you carry. After all, your total weight reflects a composite of tissue, organs, skeleton, water, and clothing. Traditional strategies for ensuring a more pleasing result of weighing are to take off your shoes or urinate before you step onto the scale. In fact, we've seen desperate people cut their fingernails, take off jewelry, strip naked, and actually stand on tiptoes! These tricks may fool the scale into registering a lighter you, but the simple truth is that your fat content will not change. You are what you are.

Determining your body composition will require the assistance of a health care professional using skin-fold calipers or a high-tech electronic measuring device, but you can get a general idea about whether you are fat (at risk) or lean (less at risk) by calculating your Body Mass Index (BMI), a ratio between your height and weight, a formula that correlates with body fat. The four-step procedure is:

1. Multiply your weight in pounds by 703.

2. Multiply your height in inches by your height in inches.

3. Divide the answer in step 1 by the answer in step 2 to get your BMI.

4. Round that number off.

Here's an example of the calculation for a person 5'5" tall and weighing 149 pounds:

1. Multiply your weight in pounds by 703: $149 \times 703 = 104,747$.

2. Multiply your height in inches by your height in inches: $65" \times 65" = 4,225"$.

3. Divide the answer in step 1 by the answer in step 2 to get your BMI: $104,747 \div 4,225 = 24.8$.

4. Round that number off: The person's BMI is 25.

Here's what your calculated BMI means:

BMI Category	Health Risk Based on BMI
Less than 25	Minimal
25–<27	Low
27–<30	Moderate
30–<35	High
35–<40	Very high
More than 40	Extremely high

Where you carry your weight is important, too. "Apple"-shaped people, who carry their weight around their waistline, are at greater risk of weight-related disease than "pear"-shaped people, who carry their weight in their hips, buttocks, and thighs. It is simple to determine your body type. If your waist is almost the same size as your hips or larger than your hips, you are an "apple" and need to get to work to reduce your body fat.

MANAGING CALORIES WITHOUT SKIMPING ON NUTRITION

Planning an athlete's diet doesn't mean that you must give up food. It means only that you make better choices and control portions more intelligently. Eating is one of life's greatest pleasures, and that doesn't have to change when you adjust your menus to include healthy foods. In fact, you should enjoy your food MORE, knowing that you're getting healthier with every bite and you're fueling your training.

A good guide for planning your diet is the U.S. Food and Drug Administration's Food Pyramid shown on page 214.

The Food Pyramid suggests that grains, fruits, and vegetables should be the foundation of your eating plan. On top of that, you may add moderate amounts of lean meats and low-fat or nonfat dairy products. In even smaller amounts, you may consume fats, oils, and sweets (including alcohol), which are high in calories and low in nutritional value.

Variety is the spice of life *and* the key to successful diet planning. The USDA suggests that you should choose different foods from each

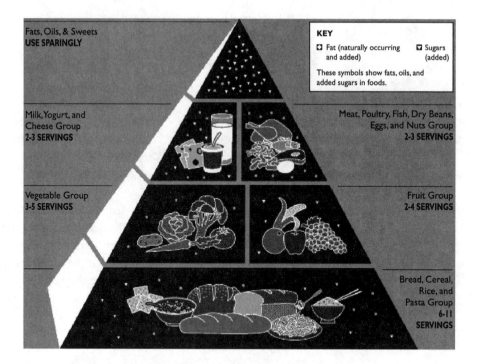

group daily and eat a variety. (And, no, chocolate is NOT a food group, in spite of what you've heard.)

TIPS ON SETTING YOUR TRAINING TABLE

1. Choose Foods Low in Fat, Saturated Fat, and Cholesterol

Your first step is to begin reading food labels. Then use that information to keep your intake of fat grams under 30 percent of the total calories you consume in a day. It is a simple matter of replacing fatty foods with less fatty foods. Let's assume that you have determined that you perform best by consuming 2,200 calories a day. Following this general guideline, you could calculate 30 percent of the 2,200 calories and set your goal: "I will consume no more than 660 calories of fat a day." There are 9 calories in a gram of fat. Dividing those calories by 9 will tell you that you should eat no more than approximately 73 grams of fat per day.

A study at Pennsylvania State University identified techniques that were effective in achieving a diet with less than 30 percent of total calories from fat. Because higher-fat meats and whole milk are the sources for a large percentage of fat in the American diet, the researchers targeted these foods for replacement with lower-fat substitutes. They discovered that simple, modest changes were easier for their participating dieters to handle—and more effective in achieving dietary goals—than trying to totally give up chips, cookies, and occasional treats. The work demonstrated that, when you decrease fat in the diet, you automatically decrease calories. A person can lose between one-half to one pound per week just by decreasing fat from a theoretical present average level of 36 percent of calories to the recommended level of 30 percent. Even women in the study, because they had low calorie-intake requirements and each food choice represents a larger proportion of the diet, lost weight most effectively by using combinations of simple changes that included replacing whole milk with skim milk, replacing high-fat meats with lean meats, and replacing full-fat products with fat-modified products.

The Penn State researchers stressed that, "By making simple changes, men and women can meet dietary goals for both total fat and saturated fat without depriving themselves of some of the higher-fat foods they enjoy."

Don't interpret "low-fat" and "fat-free" as a license to eat as much as you want. You can eat totally fat-free and take in whopping caloric counts. On the other hand, while calories count, be careful not to go too low. The fewer the calories, the more difficult it is to meet your daily requirements for nutrients to maintain good health.

A word about cholesterol. We used to regard cholesterol as a man's problem. Not any more. Women tend to have natural high levels of HDL cholesterol (the "good" cholesterol) until menopause, when researchers suspect there is a link between diminishing HDLs and diminishing estrogen levels. Vigilance is important throughout life, but it becomes critical in your middle years, when a diet high in saturated fat and cholesterol can be dangerous. For both men *and* women, it is best to keep blood cholesterol levels below 200 mg/dl. Two ways to do that are: (1) limit food from animal sources—such as egg yolks, dairy products, meat, poultry, and shellfish; and (2) reduce your intake of saturated fat.

2. *Limit Your Serving Sizes*

How much food is enough and how much is too much? It's a question best answered with a calculator and a pencil. One good way to take control of your eating habits and learn about portion control is to keep a little food diary for a couple of days. Record what you eat, when you eat it, and why. You'll quickly learn a lot about your habits and, with your calculator and pencil, you'll be able to spot some mistakes you might not be aware you're making. You'll discover that, with careful planning, you can still have all your favorite foods—in moderation. For example, a three-ounce portion of meat (roughly the size of a deck of cards) is considered to be a standard serving.

3. *Get Off the Couch*

Simply put, move it *and* lose it. In a study recently released by the North American Association for the Study of Obesity, researchers report that getting the weight off and, more important, keeping it off were successful with programs that included healthy eating combined with vigorous aerobic exercise. Exercising for thirty minutes three times a week turns up your metabolic "thermostat," helping you to burn calories. And more good news: You will continue to burn calories at an accelerated rate for hours after your workout. Muscles burn fat, so replacing body fat with lean, strong muscles gives you an even greater ability to burn calories. But regular physical activity does more than help you lose weight. It makes you feel and look better, helps lower high blood pressure and cholesterol, and can reduce your risk of cardio-vascular disease.

You don't have to join a gym to exercise aerobically. You can put on a pair of good shoes and go for a brisk walk. Or you can swim, bike, run, or dance around your living room. Start slowly and work up to a comfortable pace. Be certain to check with your physician before you begin any new exercise program, to make certain that it is safe for you. See Part III, Coaches' Notes (pp. 105–189) for a quick guide to all the fun you can have.

4. *Limit Your Sodium Intake*

A low-sodium diet can help reduce your risk of developing high blood pressure, heart and vascular disease, and kidney disease. Reducing your intake of salt-cured and smoked foods, such as hot dogs and pickles, appears to lower your risk of stomach cancer. Also, salt can cause your body to excrete calcium in your urine. You need to stay in positive calcium balance to protect your bones from osteoporosis as you get older. Take the salt shaker off the table. Use herbs and spices in your cooking instead of salt. And avoid processed and fast foods, which are usually high in sodium (and fat, as well).

5. Increase Complex Carbohydrates

The Food Pyramid suggests a solid foundation based on complex carbo-hydrates. Those are found in breads, cereals, rice, pasta, crackers, and other baked goods made from *whole grains* that are nutrient-rich. If the suggested six to seven servings a day sounds like a lot, realize that one slice of bread, a half-cup of cooked cereal or pasta, or one cup of ready-to-eat cereal equals one serving. A sandwich is two full servings.

6. Increase Dietary Fiber

A fiber-rich diet is helpful in management of healthy digestion and may be related to lower rates of colon cancer. Fiber comes in two forms—soluble and insoluble. Insoluble fiber, found primarily in whole grains, fruits, and vegetables, provides bulk for the formation of stools and helps move wastes more quickly through the colon. Soluble fiber is found in peas and beans, many vegetables and fruits, and rice, corn, and oat bran, and has been linked to lowering blood cholesterol levels. Good ways to get fiber into your diet are to eat fruit (don't peel apples, peaches, plums, or pears), add cooked beans and peas to soups and salads, use whole wheat flour whenever possible, eat whole-grain foods, use brown rice instead of white, eat low-fat bran muffins instead of plain, and snack on washed fruits and vegetables.

7. Eat Enough Calcium

Osteoporosis is the thinning of bone and is a direct result of calcium de-ficiency. Although the problem actually begins earlier in life, osteoporo-sis is defined as a major health risk in middle and later years, particularly in postmenopausal women. Calcium is used for maintaining bone struc-ture and for slowing down the loss of calcium from bones. It's best to get calcium from foods rather than supplements, so you will need to eat at least two to three servings of calcium-rich food a day. Select low-fat or skim milk, low-fat or nonfat yogurt, low-fat cheeses, canned fish with bones, green and leafy vegetables, and dried beans and peas. A special note for women: Experts recommend that all women in midlife consume at least 1,000 milligrams of elemental calcium per day if you are premenopausal, 1,200 milligrams per day if you are perimenopausal, and 1,400 milligrams per day if you are postmenopausal. If you are unable to get enough calcium from your food, you must take supplements. Talk to your doctor to get recommendations.

8. Eat Enough Iron

Although iron is important for both men and women, women tend to be deficient. Before menopause, the Recommended Dietary Allowance (RDA) for iron is 15 milligrams a day for women (as opposed to only 10 milligrams for men). This increased need in women is due to the loss of 15–20 milligrams of iron each month during menstruation. After menopause, the incidence of iron deficiency diminishes due to the cessation of menstruation, although women still need to keep a watch on iron. Low levels may indicate blood loss that is not apparent or iron-deficiency anemia, characterized by pallor, fatigue, and headaches. There are two good sources of dietary iron: *heme* from animal products, and *non-heme* found in peas, beans, spinach, green leafy vegetables, potatoes, and whole-grain and iron-fortified cereal products. Note that the addition of small amounts of vitamin C in your food substantially increases the total amount of iron absorbed from a meal.

9. Consider Vitamin and Mineral Supplements

One of the real challenges in being an athlete is hitting the balance between satisfying your need for nutrition without loading more calories that you need. The trick is to eat enough, but not too much. Dietitians suggest (and we agree) that it's best to get all your nutrients from food, but this can be tricky. If you're consuming fewer than 2,000 calories a day, it's almost impossible to get all the nutrients you need from food—even if your meals are conscientiously planned and prepared, and are based on the Food Pyramid. You're going to come up short on some pretty important things like iron, zinc, and vitamin B_6. Some studies have found that 90 percent of all Americans think they're eating a balanced diet, and yet only 10 percent are getting the nutrients they need. Although we have RDA guidelines, they cover only 18 essential vitamins and minerals (the Big 18) needed to prevent dietary deficiency. They don't cover ALL the possibilities (and you've no doubt

Vitamins

Vitamin A and Beta Carotene

Benefits: Help in maintaining good vision, healthy skin, developing bones and teeth, and resisting infection.

Food sources: Liver, egg yolk, leafy green vegetables, deep yellow/orange vegetables, sweet potatoes, and apricots.

B Vitamin Group

Benefits: Help turn food into energy, maintain a healthy nervous system, and produce red blood cells.

Food sources: Whole grains, meat, fish, poultry, legumes, and dairy products.

Vitamin C

Benefits: Helps in healing wounds, utilization of iron, healthy teeth and gums, and fighting infection.

Food sources: Citrus fruit and juice, strawberries, cantaloupe, tomatoes, broccoli, green vegetables, and potatoes.

Vitamin D

Benefits: Helps body to use calcium to build strong bones and teeth.

Food sources: Milk, egg yolk, fish oils. NOTE: Sunlight on your skin activates vitamin D.

Vitamin E

Benefits: Prevents damage to cells by protecting them from free radicals, assists healing, protects vitamins A and C from being attacked.

Food sources: Vegetable oils, avocados, wheat germ oil, nuts, margarine, legumes.

Minerals

Iron

Benefits: Assists in production of energy-rich blood.

Food sources: Liver, meats, green leafy vegetables, whole grains. NOTE: Vitamin C assists in absorption.

Calcium

Benefits: Helps build strong bones and teeth.

Food sources: Dairy products, sardines, greens, broccoli, legumes.

(Continued)

Phosphorous

Benefits: Works with calcium to help build strong bones and teeth.

Food sources: Dairy products, egg yolk, meat, poultry, fish, whole grains, nuts, and legumes.

Sodium and Potassium

Benefits: Assist in maintaining fluid balances in your body, important for muscle contraction and nerve transmission.

Food sources: Potassium is found in fruits, dairy products, cereals, vegetables, and legumes. Sodium is found in processed foods and table salt.

Iodine

Benefits: Helps form hormones that control metabolism.

Food sources: Iodized salt, saltwater fish, oysters.

Zinc and Magnesium

Benefits: Assist normal growth and development, and bodily functions.

Food sources: Almost all foods.

discovered, as we have, that there are mind-boggling lists of supplementary nutrients). And the RDA guidelines don't address the possible benefits of exceeding the minimum amounts of the Big 18. When you work out and put your body under stress, you might require more than minimum amounts of something. But what? Our best advice is to consult a licensed, registered dietitian who specializes in working with athletes, or ask your physician about vitamin and mineral supplements. Be careful about self-prescribing. Don't overdose vitamins. In large doses, some vitamins are toxic. And remember, taking vitamins and minerals isn't a substitute for eating food. You still need to sit down to a good training table meal.

10. Drink Plenty of Fluids

Water is an important part of every healthy diet, but as an athlete your requirements are enormous. (You ARE sweating, aren't you? Good! We thought so.) Drinking eight to ten large glasses of water a day will help avoid dehydration. If you wish, you might use sports drinks especially designed for athletes. They're made to replace not only fluid, but sugars, salts, minerals, and electrolytes. Be aware of their contents and their calories. Staying adequately hydrated also assists digestion and kidney function, and will help control constipation.

11. Break the Caffeine Habit

Caffeine is a powerful central nervous system stimulant found in hundreds of foods, beverages, and drugs. You may now be using it to feel more alert, but there are compelling reasons for considering cutting back. Caffeine interferes with calcium absorption, and you need a positive balance in calcium to guard against osteoporosis. In addition, caffeine acts as a diuretic and may overload the bladder with urine, triggering or exacerbating urinary incontinence (loss of bladder control). For women in postmenopausal and later years, hot flashes and other uncomfortable symptoms may interfere with sleep. Caffeine makes it more difficult to fall asleep, decreases the time you stay asleep, and diminishes the quality of sleep. To cut down, switch to decaffeinated versions of your favorite beverages. If you have been a heavy drinker of caffeine and you quit cold turkey, you can expect some withdrawal symptoms such as irritability, nervousness, restlessness, lethargy, nausea, and headaches. Get tough and hang in there! They're temporary. To lessen any symptoms of withdrawal, cut back gradually. Now that we've told you to cut back on caffeine, let us tell you about one instance when you might want to consider pouring it on. Caffeine frees fatty acids in the blood and makes energy available to fuel an endurance workout. Many marathon runners and long-distance cyclists will down a cup of coffee right before a workout, to get an extra "edge." The actual benefits of this are a little controversial, but you might want to try it to see whether it makes a difference in your performance. If it works at all, we would think you would realize the best effect if your overall caffeine levels are low. We're still advising you to cut back or eliminate caffeine from your diet.

Healthy diet and a healthy life go hand in hand, especially for an athlete. Making intelligent choices and mapping out an intelligent strategy for food selection, preparation, and consumption give you some effective controls over your well-being. Taking charge of your body often begins with taking charge of your grocery list. Remember that small changes make big differences in balancing the scales toward a healthy diet.

Finding a Qualified Dietitian

If you have a hard time making changes in your diet, you might consider working with a registered, licensed dietitian. These are health care professionals trained and uniquely qualified to work in concert with your physician to (1) evaluate your present medical status, (2) help you set goals, and (3) assist in planning and implementation of your new eating plan. Select a dietician who specializes in *Sports Nutrition.* Ask your physician for a referral, contact a local university nutrition department, look in the Yellow Pages of your phone book, or request a list of qualified registered dietitians in your area from: American Dietetic Association, 216 West Jackson Boulevard, Suite 800, Chicago, Illinois, 60606-6995.

That Voodoo That You Do

ENHANCING PERFORMANCE

When you have worked in sports as long as we have, you get to see a lot of performance-enhancement practices. In those final moments, when an athlete steps up to put it all on the line, we've seen rituals and behaviors that run the gamut from carrying voodoo dolls to drinking the water from boiled maize. Forget science and statistics. Forget biology, physiatry, physiology, physics, genetics, dietetics, kinetics, and coaching. All that stuff fades into distant memory in the searing glare of the task at hand. At this moment, the athlete's job is to galvanize training and desire into one exquisitely laser-focused moment. This consolidation has to be greater than the sum of its parts. Something has to bring it all together and make it work. We have always known that there is something mystical in an athlete's spirit that makes it possible to harness power. When an athlete reaches in and marshals that intangible, ephemeral "something," he or she performs at levels beyond personal capability. Although these "super" performances astonish us, we are seldom surprised. We have long known and respected athletes' magic. If wearing purple underwear or kissing a coach's bald head is the key that locks the formula into place, then it has our blessing.

In this chapter, we are discussing performance-enhancing practices without judgment (the exceptions being drugs and chemicals). In some cases, however, we reserve the right to laugh hysterically in private.

WHAT TO WEAR

Wearing a uniform or special outfit has two purposes. First, it's practical. Shoes and clothing have been designed to meet the specifications of each sport and assist the athlete in performance. For example, running shorts are made of fabric as light as butterfly wings. They wick sweat straight off the body and allow the skin to breathe and cool. The side panels of the shorts legs are split, allowing full, unimpeded range of motion for pumping legs. In some shorts, there's a lining that supports the runner. On the other hand, cycling shorts are engineered to fit tightly so that the cyclist won't snag on things at roadside. The shorts hug the leg to the mid-thigh, to protect the skin from scraping and to eliminate wind resistance. The seat, crotch, and inner thighs are lightly padded to protect the fanny from the pressure of the cycle seat.

The second purpose of a special outfit is to create an identity with the sport. Theoretically, when you dress like an athlete, it's easier to BE an athlete. Don't laugh. We've seen a lot of workouts trashed when athletes had to borrow clothing or "make do" with clothing that was not sport-specific. Perhaps the clothing was not as functional as it should have been, but you'll never convince us that part of the problem wasn't a sudden lack of confidence, a sudden disassociation with serious commitment to the sport. On the flip side, we've seen lackluster performance levels rocketed after a trip to the local sporting goods store. We gave an inexpensive runner's watch to a friend who was just beginning running and on the verge of quitting. With that watch on her wrist, suddenly she felt like a runner and started training like one. Little things can make big differences.

Let us give you one inside tip about clothing. There's something squeaky and desperate about totally brand-new clothes in sports. Don't let anyone see you wearing clothing or shoes straight out of the bag. Wash your stuff first. New clothes shout, "BEGINNER!" You don't want to feel that way.

Sunglasses

Many athletes wear sunglasses not only to protect their eyes, but to prevent competitors from seeing their eyes. There is something cool and aloof about a person whose eyes are masked. If you really want to unhinge competitors, wear reflective lenses. Not only will they be unable to see your eyes, but they will see only their own concerned, alarmed reflection. If you want to complete the intimidation, wear wraparounds. They completely block off your eyes and appear to be aerodynamic—unsettling proof that you intend to be moving so quickly that you'll need to minimize wind resistance and protect your face from windburn. If you wear sunglasses when you participate in physical activity, make sure they're UV-screening and shatterproof, and offer protection from impact.

Hair

Most sports have a "look" that is reflected in hairstyles. These styles are evolved from practical function, but many develop into signatures of the sport. Braids for skiing. Short pony tails for gymnastics. Shaved heads for swimming. Short, with a painter's cap, for marathon running. Again, styling is one more way to create an identity with the sport. Theoretically, if you look like an athlete, you'll perform like an athlete.

Lucky Charms

A piece of clothing sometimes becomes an object of superstition. A pair of socks that were worn during a winning event might suddenly become necessary for any win. They become "lucky." The athlete will not compete without them. Also, sometimes clothing becomes familiar and comforting. A favorite singlet, for example, might make an athlete feel better when the pressure is on.

RITUALS

Rituals are methodical practices that must be performed before the athlete can step up to the line. No matter how ridiculous a ritual might seem to the outside observer, if the athlete isn't allowed to perform the ritual, disaster will follow. One of our friends volunteered to work at a small track meet and was assigned to security on the outside field at the third turn on the far side of the track. When it was over, we apologized for encouraging her to volunteer and promising her the excitement of a real track meet, and we expressed regret that she wasn't assigned near the start and finish line, where all the action takes place. She said, "Are you kidding? That far corner is where all the runners sneak away to prepare for their races. I've never seen such bizarre behavior in my life! It was incredibly entertaining!" What she had observed were the rituals. One of the more common ones is simple praying. Others include such things as touching "lucky" objects, performing ceremonies, packing equipment or putting on clothing in a certain order, singing special songs, and chanting. Rituals are used to focus the mind, to harness energy, to calm nerves, to engage in mindless activity as a way of quieting the chaos of the competition, and to invite assistance from the cosmos. We've seen some pretty odd things, but we never question their purposes. We understand completely.

If you notice another athlete performing a ritual, the rule of thumb is: "Don't join in." Also, don't break into hysterical laughter, point, or call others over to "see this." In fact, don't even watch. If you find yourself slipping into rituals, select discreet practices. We don't want to see you smearing chicken blood on your coach.

TOKENS

Athletes, in their quest for mojo, often will collect objects that help them win. We've seen four-leaf clovers, rabbits' feet, horseshoes, crystals, angels, medallions, pins, earrings, rings, brooches, dolls, teddy bears and other stuffed animals, clothing and equipment from other champion athletes, blankets, towels, religious medals, keys—you name it and we've seen it. These tokens are carried in the clothing of the athlete, worn as jewelry, or tucked into a secret corner of a gear bag. Even the most logical, rational, mature athlete is likely to have a little "something" magical that represents winning. Again, if you find yourself gravitating toward a token, select the right one. Choose something small and unlikely to attract attention. A lucky airplane propeller might seem like a good idea at the time, but your fellow athletes will think you're nuts.

ABSTINENCE

Some athletes believe that making love before a competition will sap the body of vital energy and guarantee an abysmal performance. The legends of sports are rife with stories of celibacy and sacrifice. One of the Olympic compendiums contains a wonderful anecdote about Bob Beamon, an Olympic gold medalist in the long jump. It reports that on the night before the most important final contest in his career, Bob Beamon did something he had never done before: he made love on the night before a major competition. He immediately regretted it and became overwhelmed with dread that he had just blown his one shot at the world record that he had boasted he would win. Good-bye, Olympic Gold! He needn't have worried. The next day was a triumph. When officials verified his score, Beamon was so relieved that he collapsed.*

Experts who have studied the practice of abstinence (we would like to see how they word THESE surveys!) conclude that there is no statistical or biological evidence that making love the night before an athletic event has any effect on performance. Nor does abstaining. Apparently, it's a matter of individual choice.

DRUGS

As benevolently as we support performance-enhancing practices, we absolutely draw the line at chemicals and drugs. Under NO circumstances should any athlete use chemicals or drugs at any time. Period.

Here's what the International Olympic Committee has to say:

> Although the subject received unprecedented attention, the use of performance-enhancing drugs is not new. There are those who say that all performance-enhancing drugs should be legalized, that drug users will always stay one step away from the testers (masking). However, the harmful side effects of banned substances, steroids specifically, justifies vigilance.

If an athlete is dying to win, there's no better way than to load up on steroids. Testosterone and its over forty identified synthetic derivatives have a chemical structure that is both anabolic (protein building) and androgenic (masculinizing). Anabolic steroids are manufactured in pill form (short metabolic half-lives), or as an oil-based diluent that must be injected (long metabolic half-lives and slow tissue release). Under optimum circumstances, the use of anabolic steroids increases

---

*The Complete Book of the Olympics by David Wallechinsky. (1991). Little, Brown & Company: Canada.

Anabolic Steroids Aren't the Only Culprits

The United States Olympic Committee (USOC) has set a gold standard for prohibited substances and methods. A great number of things can enhance performance. If an athlete tests positively for any of them, he or she is in big trouble—in more ways than one.

Doping Classes

- *Stimulants,* including a shocking array of over-the-counter medications you can find in your local pharmacy; caffeine; and some asthma medications.
- *Narcotic analgesics,* including some common, mild, prescription pain killers.
- *Testosterone,* in excess in men and women (unless the presence of excessive testosterone can be explained by a physiological or pathological condition).
- *Other anabolic agents,* such as growth hormones.

Doping Methods

- *Blood doping,* defined as the intravenous transfusion of red blood cells or related blood products that contain red blood cells.
- *Pharmacological, chemical, and physical manipulation.* Tampering with a urine sample.

Substances Subject to Certain Restrictions

- *Alcohol, marijuana, local anesthetics.*

Corticosteroids

- *Substances found mostly in anti-inflammatory drugs that relieve pain.* Forbidden except for topical use, inhalation therapy, and local or intra-articular injections.

Beta Blockers

- *Substances used for control of high blood pressure, cardiac arrhythmias, angina pectoris, and migraine headaches.* These may or may not be allowed, depending on medical recommendations.

If you have questions, call the USOC Hotline at 1–800–233–0393.

protein synthesis, lean body mass, and nitrogen balance. Unfortunately, there have been few credible clinical trials to test the effectiveness of anabolic steroids in strength training and body building, so most of what we know about any benefits has been anecdotal. Even more unfortunately, there is little chance that we will ever know more. Because anabolic steroids have proved themselves to be deadly and are illegal, clinical trials in the United States would violate medical ethics and law. If we're to learn more about anabolic steroids, that information is going to have to come from studies elsewhere in the world. Although we can't test anabolic steroids, we can test *for* them. And we do. When an athlete competes in an event sanctioned or governed by the sport or by an organization like the International Olympic Committee (IOC), you can bet that he or she will be tested. If the results are positive, the consequences are severe. The purpose in suspending or banning an athlete is not to punish. It's to save his or her life. Sports officials think that if the athlete no longer feels the pressure of competition, perhaps he or she will no longer take steroids.

The use of anabolic steroids is harmful to the liver and to the reproductive, endocrine, cardiovascular, musculoskeletal, and central nervous systems. (Is there ANYTHING left?) The deterioration, damage, and disease caused by anabolic steroids can all have a common side effect: death.

Over the years, we have had clients march us into health food stores and press our faces into shelves of pills, powders, and potions that claim all sorts of wonderful things. Let's have a moment of truth here. If health and fitness were as easy as mixing up a shake, we would all be doing it. There may be benefit to some products, but there are no miracles out there. You're being lied to when you read the label of newly discovered, cutting-edge, breakthrough, formerly secret Tibetan, herbal, mineral, vitamin-packed, protein-charged, oxygenated, low-calorie, fat-free, algae-laced powder. If you eat a healthy, balanced diet based on sound principles, you'll do great! Leave the fancy stuff to the people who try to buy fitness rather than work for it.

It's a Jungle Out There

Here's a question for you. Which athlete will be more successful—one who trains with a group or one who trains at home alone? If you assumed that success is guaranteed to a person who seeks safety in numbers and relies on group support as a valuable incentive for staying with a fitness program, you would be wrong. Recently released studies indicate that the athlete who works out alone does better! Of course, everyone is different and many people prefer the security, regimentation, and discipline of a group workout. But if you decide to stay at home, statistics are in your favor. You'll do well.

Getting fit has never been easier with equipment and programs specifically designed for home use. You can work out in the comfort, safety, and privacy of your own home and at your convenience. You don't need to drive any distance or wear fancy outfits. You don't have to pay fitness club membership fees. You don't have to wait in line to use equipment during peak hours. As an extra bonus, equipment at home can be enjoyed by family members and friends. And there are lots of good choices. But it's a jungle out there. Making a few decisions and gathering information *before* you begin shopping can save you time, spare you difficulty, and get you off to a good start on your personal fitness program.

TYPES OF EQUIPMENT YOU CAN BUY

These are the five basic types of home gym equipment:

1. *Variable resistance weight training equipment.* Most often, these are the machines that operate with such devices as pulleys, cams, weights, and counterbalances. They are commonly associated with trendy fitness centers.

2. *Cardiovascular equipment* is designed to get your heart rate up and give you a good aerobic workout. Bikes, ski machines, stair steppers, and treadmills are in this category.

3. *Free weights* are basic dumbbells and barbells, called "free" because they are attached to nothing (except you.)

4. *Hybrid equipment* is designed to combine one or more functions—usually cardiovascular and variable resistance weight training. A good example of a hybrid would be a stationary bike with arm pulls or a "rider" that requires you to crunch up your abdomen and pull the handlebars toward you in order to get it to move.

5. *Toys,* or sporting equipment for you to play with.

With so many choices in designing your home gym and choosing your equipment, the keys to success are: setting your personal goals, defining your personal style, setting aside a space, and deciding how much money you have to spend.

LAYING THE GROUNDWORK FOR YOUR HOME GYM

Getting back into shape, getting into shape for the first time, or augmenting the fitness program you already have in place requires some careful thought. The first step always, in stepping into a fitness program, is to consult your physician. Most physicians today are great advocates of exercise. They recognize its undeniable benefits with regard to your health and well-being. You may be surprised pleasantly to find yourself being offered an "exercise prescription"—complete with a program, guidelines, and an enthusiastic endorsement.

You need to be clear about what you wish to accomplish. We support a "total" approach to getting fit.

After you set your goals, you need to define your style. The best equipment in the world does you no good if you will not use it. (We know lots of people who drape their laundry over stationary bikes.) You have to be able to handle the equipment, and to integrate the program into your life and your home. Most important, the home gym you design and the program you develop have to be fun for you.

Space is an important consideration in designing your home gym. A single piece of home gym equipment can take up as little as ten square inches or as much as a hundred square feet. And you might decide to invest in more than one piece of equipment. If it isn't practical to put your home gym outside or build a separate room for it, survey your home to find a space that you are willing to give up (with a little furniture rearranging). Many people select a corner of the bedroom or den. These tend to be private, family-only rooms where the decor is not so important that the introduction of exercise equipment will be inappropriate. Additionally, it's fun to put the equipment in the "middle of things" where it is likely to be used. Many people like to locate their equipment in front of a television set. They can then enjoy programs and videotapes for motivation or distraction while they work out. (We advise caution to those of you who might be overly enthusiastic and plant yourself in front of the tube with your family across the room behind you, craning their necks and jockeying for position to see over your shoulder. It strains relations, big time.) You might enjoy positioning your equipment in front of windows so you can look outside, or in front of a poster of a competitor so you can remember why you're training and whom you have to beat. Music is always a big favorite. (But make sure you pop in something with an energetic beat. Nothing kills a workout like a funeral dirge.) An interesting report put out by ACE FitnessMatters advises that watching TV for thirty minutes while exercising will decrease your intensity by 5 percent as opposed to listening to music (which will increase your intensity). Upbeat music will increase your intensity without increasing your level of perceived exertion—IF you like the music. Magazine and book racks, in an adequately lighted area, can help turn your workout into a double-duty activity as you catch up on reading while training. (If you're checking out library books, be particularly careful. Nothing annoys a librarian like a soggy novel.) Because working out causes your body to heat up, you'll want a portable fan to use, in addition to normal air-conditioning. Sweat might ruin your good carpet (we're assuming that you'll sweat!), so you'll want to put a protective pad or inexpensive area rug under your equipment. Electricity can be a factor if your equipment of choice requires power, so you need to survey the availability of outlets. And experts agree that positioning a mirror (the bigger the better!) is helpful in checking on and maintaining your proper form. Under some circumstances, the harsh reality of a mirror could also serve as an incentive to work a little harder.

Decide how much money you're willing to spend. A single piece of home gym equipment can range in price from under $100 to over $7,000. Experts warn that "expensive" is not necessarily "better," so you'll want to shop carefully. Think of the money you spend as an investment in yourself, and use it as a motivator for sticking with your program, but don't waste it. Experts advise you to always insist on a money-back guarantee and a good warranty. Be cautious when shopping from a catalog or ordering from your computer or television. Nothing beats a hands-on demonstration to decide whether a piece of equipment is for you. If you are purchasing sight-unseen, guarantees and warranties are doubly important.

Most home gym equipment comes unassembled and you'll need to put it together when it arrives. Many retailers are glad to send an installer to assist you (for an additional fee). If you decide to assemble it alone, find out (in advance!) how complicated the assembly is and what tools you need. Also, remember that some home gym equipment is heavy (particularly after it is assembled) and you may need some help in getting it into position.

WHAT TO LOOK FOR IN LIFTING EQUIPMENT

We have offered you everything you need to put together a good strength program, but there will always be a few among us who aren't happy unless there's a gleaming, clanging, padded machine occupying most of the floor space in the den. If you want to get really fancy, you can install *variable resistance weight training* equipment, which uses cables or pulleys connected to a stack of heavy metal weights that are kept in line by a vertical bar or track. The weights provide "resistance" against which you push or pull. This resistance is called "variable" because you adjust it to be heavier or lighter as needed. Pushing and pulling against this resistance strengthens your muscles. For the most part, the newer variable resistance weight training equipment selections are safe, often protecting your lower back and forcing you to use better form and technique. Balance and coordination are not difficult. And some equipment is designed to avoid hand gripping, which can drive blood pressure up dramatically. If the piece is well designed with a number of functions integrated into its use, you can get a good strength workout. Although cables and pulleys are used most commonly, rubber bands, flexible rods, shock absorbers, and/or centrifugal brakes also may be used to provide resistance. Although no system seems to be better than another at helping you build muscles, each has a different "feel" and you should try each to find the one that is best for you. Look for equipment that is well constructed and comfortable. Keep in mind: while you are getting a good workout, so is your equipment. Make certain that you select a piece that will last a long time and do a good job for you. Inspect the joints and look for bent or welded metal rather than bolted. Seat upholstery, hand grips, pads, and handles should be constructed of heavy materials and be covered under the warranty. Be sure to keep the equipment clean, dry, and disinfected. These babies are hotbeds of pestilence. Are you used to having the invisible housekeeping staff of the local gym care for the equipment you use? Unless you can pay them to come over to your house, cleaning's up to you now.

WHAT TO LOOK FOR IN CARDIOVASCULAR EQUIPMENT

Studies have shown that strength training offers little significant cardiovascular benefit, so if you decide that you need an aerobic workout in your home gym routine, you should first consider buying yourself an inexpensive pair of walking or running shoes. Or dust off your bicycle. Or get into the pool. But, if you really enjoy high-tech equipment, you might invest in cardiovascular equipment such as a treadmill, ski machine, stair stepper, or bike.

Quality electric treadmills start at about $1,200 and range up to $7,000. The machine must be able to stand the strain of a regular workout and should have a continuous motor rating of over 1.5 horsepower. Each footfall of a 150-pound running person slams the belt against the running board with up to 600 pounds of pressure—effectively pinning the belt to the board for a moment, and jamming the motor. The motor must recover and continue nearly 1,000 times every mile, so a top-rated motor has to be your first consideration when selecting your equipment.

Some treadmills offer more shock absorption than others, so look for thicker running belts, thinner running decks, aluminum frames that flex more than steel, and shock absorbers. Top speeds vary. Select one that is consistent with your goals—and probably just a little faster than you will want to go, just in case you improve beyond your wildest imagination. The belt should be long and wide, so you have as much walking/running space as possible. Look for handrails that are there for safety but are not in the way of your arm swing. And consider options such as a heart rate monitor, the ability to elevate the treadmill for a simulated uphill workout, automatic cutoff if you get into trouble, and entertaining programs in the electronics, mileage calculators, and calorie counters. Nonmotorized treadmills are available with a surprising number of options. They will give you a great workout, and cost considerably less.

Exercise bikes, like treadmills, can be motorized or nonmotorized, and they come with a lot of options, some of which will help you maximize your workout and some of which will entertain you while you sweat. They are less expensive than treadmills, however, ranging in price from under $100 to over $2,000. A recent innovation in exercise bikes is the "recumbent bike," which allows you to sit in a chair-back with your feet pedaling in front of you and is easier on your lower back, arms, hands, and fanny. Both types of bikes, upright and recumbent, are equally effective in providing a good workout. Programmed or manual pedal resistance is a valuable feature, allowing you to vary your workout from a hard push up an imaginary steep hill for leg strength to a quick spin for cardiovascular fitness. Comfort is important. Make certain that you are able to adjust the seat height to fit you and that the seat affords you adequate cushioning, blister control, and sweat absorption.

Stair steppers, long a high-tech favorite of fitness-center clientele, have found their way into the home gym setting in affordable versions (priced similarly to bikes). These, like the treadmills and exercise bikes, are both motorized and nonmotorized. And both ways, they offer a good cardiovascular workout. Stair steppers approximate the action you take in climbing steps. Some machines have two steps on which you stand and pump up and down by lifting one foot and then the other. Some have continuously rotating steps that you merely "climb." And some allow you to position your feet on steps and work out on an elliptical cycle. Look for safety features such as a handrail in front and to the sides of you. A good stair stepper has options such as a heart rate monitor, variable programs, calorie counting, a timer, automatic cutoff if you get into trouble, and mileage approximation. The step surface should be nonskid.

Ski machines were developed for cross-country skiers who could ski during only one season of the year and languished unhappily during the other three. The ski machine gave them a piece of exercise equipment that helped them maintain their cardiovascular fitness and their arm and leg strength, when they couldn't get outside. Fortunately, the machine found its way into the marketplace and now a number are available ranging in price from under $500 to over $2,000. The advantages of the ski machine are: it provides a superior cardiovascular workout with no jarring to the joints; it is relatively flat so it fits into most homes; and it is nonmotorized and quiet. Many models have added an arm-workout feature. And of course, the newer models have electronic options similar to other cardiovascular equipment.

FREE WEIGHTS

Free weights are perfect for home gyms. Velcro wrist and ankle weights (such as those we use in the Active-Isolated Strength program), dumbbells (the small handheld weights), and barbells (heavy round plates fastened to each end of a metal bar) are affordable, portable, durable, blissfully low-tech, and easily stored. With free weights, each muscle is isolated and strengthened specifically.

TOYS

There's a lot to be said for the fitness benefits of toys—sporting equipment that gets you out the door to play. We're talking about toys like golf clubs, volleyballs, in-line skates, skis, and tennis racquets. Training is a means, not an end. The "end" is the reward of being fit and knowing that your body can play, that you can participate at a high level in activities that you enjoy. And trust us, fitness begets fitness. The more you play, the more fit you become.

BEWARE THE INFOMERCIAL

A word to the wise: Beware of ANY equipment manufacturer who declares that you can achieve health and fitness with no effort on your part. You'll hear hype such as, "Create rock-hard abs in just three minutes a day, three days a week!" "After one session, you'll feel ten pounds lighter and an inch taller!" "Perfect for every age and every lifestyle!" If it sounds too good to be true, it is. A study done at the Metropolitan State College of Denver on sports equipment marketing concluded that infomercials can be misleading. They can give us the impression that, if we buy and use the equipment, we'll look just like the model who's demonstrating it. Wrong. The announcer fails to mention what ELSE that model had to do to achieve that body. Although many of the manufacturers claim to deliver "total fitness," not one of them can. Fitness, as we have told you, is a multifaceted package that machines alone can't deliver. You can't assume that the people giving testimonials and representing the equipment are qualified to give you accurate information or educated opinions. They're paid, pretty people. It's the salesperson's job to get you to buy a single piece of equipment, not to give you good advice specific to your needs. Many ads make claims that are outrageous. We know it. You know it. Even they know it. But they're trading on hope, on the very human quest for "magic bullets" and easy fixes. They never tell you what risks are associated with the equipment. Their time on the air is short and their purpose is to make you salivate, dig out your charge card, and dial that phone number. If they devoted ample time to telling you all that could go wrong, you would be cowering under the couch and clutching at the channel changer. And, no matter how inexpensive advertised equipment is reported to be ("Only pennies a day!"), it's usually not a bargain. Comparison shopping at sporting goods stores, road-testing equipment for yourself, and looking for used equipment will save you aggravation and money.

No matter what you choose, the faster you see fitness results, the more likely you will stick to your program. Choosing the right equipment and then learning to use it properly are vital to effective training. We want you to hang in there!

The Older Athlete

Many things we traditionally believed to be true about the older athlete are proving to be wrong. Gone are the days when we think of growing older as a time when we creak and shuffle. As we enter our "Golden Years," we now realize that gold doesn't rust! The American Association of Retired Persons (AARP) puts it succinctly: "The experience of aging in America isn't what it used to be." No kidding. Today, with strength and flexibility training, we are more likely to dance and speedwalk. Older athletes are doing more, and more for longer, than we ever thought possible. A few modifications in training techniques and regimens must be made to accommodate an older body (particularly if the athlete is a beginner and has never worked out before). But the results are astonishing and well worth the effort. You can't turn back the hands of time, but you CAN rewind the clock.

The Sporting Goods Manufacturers Association says: "Today's 50- to 65-year-olds have much in common with younger generations. In many ways they represent the 'new youth generation,' as they comprise singles and marrieds, workers and retirees, empty nesters as well as parents with families. Most importantly, like their younger counterparts, they are looking for fun, companionship, and shared experiences. With nearly three in ten Americans aged 55 and older exercising at least 100 times a year—a higher rate than any other age group—a revolution in values and attitudes is taking place." But why stop with the 50- to 65-year-olds? An appropriate exercise program is guaranteed to be successful, no matter how old you are when you begin. One of the studies we most frequently cite when someone is whining about being too old to work out is that of Maria Fiatarone of the USDA Human Nutrition Center on Aging, at Tufts University.

Here's how Fiatarone described her findings to the House Select Committee on Aging, in February 1991:

> Starting with a small group of ten 90-year-old residents of the Hebrew Rehabilitation Center for the Aged in Massachusetts, we demonstrated that the muscle weakness and atrophy of aging were in fact not at all immutable. These residents increased their leg muscle strength by 174 percent and their muscle size by 9 percent after only eight weeks of weight-lifting exercise. More importantly, as we have expanded this research to a much larger group of volunteers through the support of grants from the National Institute of Aging and others, it is clear that such training can improve walking speeds, mobility, independence in daily activities, and reduce dependence on canes, walkers, and wheelchairs in some individuals. At a cellular level, we now have preliminary evidence that this increased muscle function is accompanied by the actual growth of new muscle fibers, a finding never before demonstrated after strength training.

Surprised that strength training was the activity of choice for these supposedly "frail" ladies and gentlemen? You shouldn't be. The late Michael Pollock, Director of the Center for Exercise Science at the University of Florida, agreed with Fiatarone. His studies on human performance demonstrate conclusively that strength training should be the cornerstone for every fitness program, and most particularly those of older people. He says that strength is the foundation of all other activity. We couldn't agree more!

And just in case you're wondering what "activity" would interest a senior athlete, the U.S. National Senior Sports Organization has in its record books stellar competitive performances in archery, bowling, cycling, golf, race walking, road racing (running), swimming, discus, high jump, javelin, long jump, pole vault, shot put, triathlon, and track and field at 100, 200, 400, 800, and 1,500 meters. Astronaut John Glenn heads back into space at age 77. Former U.S. President George Bush skydives out of an airplane at age 72. Catholic Sister Madonna Buder, born in 1930 and living in Spokane, Washington, is blithely setting Iron Man world records. (An Iron Man is a megatriathlon—a three-phase event consisting of a 2.4-mile swim, a 112-mile bike ride, and a 26.2-mile run.) Sister Madonna says matter-of-factly, "I guess I'm not ready to be put out to pasture yet." Clearly aging isn't for wimps.

The senior fitness industry might be experiencing a boom because the Baby Boomers are reaching "that age" when body parts are threatening to drift, and reality is setting in (somewhere along the hip line, we think). Some are entering the "senior" sport scene, merely continuing a lifelong commitment to fitness. Many of the athletes we work with are former Olympians and world champions who are getting older and are delighted to be regarded now as "masters." They say it's fun to shatter the records! But many other older people are starting to work out for the first time. It's never too late to begin. And there are compelling reasons to start *today*.

WE WANT TO SCARE YOU TO DEATH TO SAVE YOUR LIFE

Not only will exercise add to the quality of your life, but it might prolong it. Dr. Michael Pollock referred to a 1992 study published in *Circulation,* the journal of the American Heart Association, which elevated physical inactivity from a minor to a major health risk. Sitting on one's duff is now on the "Killer List," along with smoking, cholesterol, and hypertension. Even the U.S. Surgeon General's office has issued a terrifying warning: "The Surgeon General has determined that the lack of physical activity is detrimental to your health." (Maybe we could print this on a warning label that we could attach to couches.) In a longitudinal study conducted by Steven N. Blair, Director of Research at the Cooper Institute for Aerobic Research in Dallas, scientists followed and examined 7,080 women and 25,341 men. According to Blair, people who are sedentary have twice the risk of dying early as compared with those who are moderately fit. In fact, Blair says, "Low fitness is one of the most powerful predictors of early mortality . . . and just about doubles your risk of dying of cardiovascular disease." And the *Journal of the American Medical Association* reports a study demonstrating that low fitness is as strong a risk factor for dying as smoking. Male and female smokers who had high blood pressure or high cholesterol levels, but were moderately fit, lived longer than healthy nonsmokers who were sedentary. Blair's study confirms this. His results conclude that the most fit people who smoked and had elevated blood pressure and cholesterol, for instance, were half as likely to die as nonsmoking people who were sedentary.

The message is clear. One key to long and healthy life is to get off your duff! NOW!

EXERCISE IS THE BEST KEPT ANTIAGING SECRET AROUND

Granted, the older body experiences some changes, and some of those changes diminish physical capabilities and athletic performance. Natural aging appears to coincide with a slow loss of muscle mass—about 1 percent per year after age 30. By the time you're age 70 to 80, nearly 40 percent of your muscle mass may be gone—UNLESS, experts say, you've exercised. Since the early 1970s, Dr. Pollock followed the lives of 27 elite distance runners, walkers, and sprinters. All had placed in the top three in regional or national competitions. Now, twenty years later, the group ranges in age from 60 to 92. Ten of them are still competing in regional or national meets. "You can learn a lot from them," Dr. Pollock said. "While their upper body muscle mass appears to be shrinking, the lower level is being maintained. So it's good evidence for the importance of a well-rounded program for total body fitness." For life. Clearly, exercise might be the best kept antiaging secret around.

You need all the muscle you can get, and you need to keep it as long as you can! Muscles are like furnaces that burn fat for energy. When muscle mass diminishes, the body can't burn fat as efficiently, literally becoming less lean and more fat. This combination forms a sort of "Catch-22": less muscle means more fat, which means even less muscle, which means even more fat, which means—you get the picture. By the time you notice that your body parts are drifting and anatomical peaks and valleys are becoming redistributed, the cycle has a firm hold on you. Unless checked, the consequences are debilitating and insidious. In the past, these declines might have been accepted as normal functions of aging, but not anymore. Research and experience clearly have demonstrated that we can stay healthier in our later years by engaging in a fitness program.

IF YOU'VE BEEN AN ATHLETE ALL YOUR LIFE

In competition sports, older athletes are often "age-graded." This is a sort of handicapping system in which an athlete's age is factored into performance. Using standardized tables, achievement is compared with what it would have been in "prime" years, and adjusted according to a formula. Most sports have examined the curve—the increases in youth and the decreases in aging—and identified one peak moment when everything is optimum. This is the standard by which age-grading is measured. It's a good way to "level the playing field." We always get a kick out of seeing a masters runner crossing the finish line behind a younger runner, and winning! Here's how an age-graded track meet works. In a 100-meter race between a 34-year-old male and a 72-year-old male, officials would give the older runner a 24-meter lead. If the 72-year-old finishes 24 meters behind the younger runner, his performance would be equal (based on statistics factoring the effects of aging on human performance) to that of the young man.

Masters athletes point out that age-grading is a good way to measure your own accomplishment. Phil Mulkey, a 1960 Olympian and now a masters athlete, says that the age-graded tables for a sport have many uses, such as keeping track of your own progress over the years, setting goals based on realistic expectations, and comparing your performance against "best ever" performances—yours and those of other athletes.

To order Masters Age-Graded Tables, contact:

National Masters News Order Department
Box 50098
Eugene, OR 97405

There is a fee for the Tables, plus postage and handling. Inquire, and they'll let you know what amount to send.

FOR THE BEGINNER: THE SURGEON GENERAL HAS A PLAN TO HELP YOU GET STARTED

Exercise doesn't have to be a chore to be effective. Although we would like to have you engage in a well-rounded program that includes flexibility, strength, and cardiovascular components, the U.S. Surgeon General's office has an easy approach to getting started. They say you don't even have to break a sweat. They recommend a startlingly simple and effective exercise plan: Just burn 150 calories of extra energy a day, or 1,000 calories per week. We think this is a good way to get started on your road to fitness (as long as you swear to us that you won't stop there!). Please note that the plan suggests that you BURN 150 calories of extra energy every day rather than eliminate 150 calories from your diet.

They make a pretty good argument. By burning 150 calories of extra energy every day, you could cut your risk of heart disease by 50 percent, and reduce the risk of high blood pressure, diabetes, and colon cancer by 30 percent. The Centers for Disease Control say that exercising helps maintain healthy bones, muscles, and joints; helps control weight, build lean muscle, and reduce body fat; helps control joint swelling and pain associated with arthritis; may enhance the effect of estrogen replacement therapy in decreasing bone loss after menopause; tires you a little so you sleep better; and may help mitigate symptoms of anxiety and depression associated with aging and with menopause in women. And best of all, it will get you in the habit of engaging in activity. When you see the results, and realize how much fun you had, you'll continue.

HOW DO I BURN UP 150 CALORIES?

Moderate physical activities that could help you work off 150 calories include walking briskly for thirty minutes, swimming laps for twenty minutes, gardening for thirty to forty-five minutes, stair walking for fifteen minutes, washing and waxing a car for forty-five to sixty minutes, or pushing a stroller one mile in thirty minutes. If you can't find the time to sneak in one of these "workouts," there are studies that conclude that several short sessions are just as good as one long one, as long as they are equal in intensity. So, if you don't have the time to walk for thirty minutes, you could do it for twenty minutes and then fill in the balance with two more five-minute workouts later, when you have more time. In addition, sports medicine experts agree that, for people who are not able to set aside large blocks of time for exercise, shorter periods are better than none. And, compliance—sticking with a program—is easier when it's convenient. Welcome to real life, pal!

BURNING CALORIES MEANS LOSING WEIGHT: DOUBLE YOUR BENEFIT

Exercise means burning calories; burning calories means losing weight. You need to burn off 3,500 calories in order to lose one pound of fat. Eat your usual calories, but walk briskly each day and burn your 150 calories. In one year, you'll burn 54,750 calories, which means you'll lose 15.6 pounds. But it could get even better. Simply eat 150 fewer calories per day (lose the muffin), in addition to walking, to burn off your 150 calories. You will run a deficit of 300 calories per day and double your weight loss. You must remember that calorie expenditures vary from person to person. How much you weigh and how hard you work will determine how many calories you burn.

YOU'LL FEEL BETTER ABOUT YOURSELF

In addition to enjoying good health, one of the real advantages of your fitness program is self-esteem. With every inch you lose from your waist, every inch you gain in range of motion, every extra pound you lift, or every extra foot you walk, you will feel better about yourself. You owe it to yourself to organize a personal fitness starter program, 150 calories at a time.

HOW CAN I ENSURE THAT I WILL STAY WITH MY FITNESS PROGRAM?

Make It Safe

The Surgeon General says that previously sedentary people who begin physical activity programs should start with short intervals (five to ten minutes) of exercise and gradually build up to their desired levels. People with chronic health problems such as heart disease, diabetes, or obesity, or who are at high risk for these conditions, should first consult a physician before beginning a new program. People over age fifty who plan to begin a new program of *vigorous* physical activity should first consult a physician to be sure they do not have heart disease or other health problems.

Make It Fun

Find activities you enjoy doing and then share them with your family and friends. Exercise is not meant to be a drudgery. It is supposed to bring you joy. It's a time to play.

Make It Convenient

Fit the activity into your life as easily as you can. Do things that are easy for you to get to. If just driving to the gym takes an hour, or if your activity is equipment-intensive and requires an hour of preparation before you can work out, rethink your program.

Make It Realistic

Set goals for yourself that are realistic and attainable. Every workout will then be a success and make you feel great.

Burn Those Calories!

Estimates for a 150-Pound Person

Activity	Calories Burned in One Hour	Approximately How Long It Will Take to Burn 150 Calories
Walking	270–440	25 minutes
Tennis	400–545	20 minutes
Swimming	275–545	25 minutes
Jogging	545–740	15 minutes
Bicycling	410–545	20 minutes
Cross-country skiing	610–700	15 minutes
Running	650–920	12 minutes
Gardening	340	25 minutes
Housework	240	35 minutes
Raking leaves	270	35 minutes
Shopping	155	1 hour

WE KNOW WHAT'S BEEN STOPPING YOU—UNTIL NOW

Let's be frank. Just between us, you've been afraid. And for good reason. You don't want to look stupid. You've spent your whole life getting good at the things you know how to do. By the time you've reached that stage when you're considered "older," you're secure in your understanding of the world. You're confident. And you aren't crazy about situations where you don't know what's going on. You're really uncomfortable when you're out of control. (So far, have we got you pegged?) Jumping into fitness was jumping into a world where everything was unfamiliar. You cringed at the thought of a gym. You thought you were going to look like an idiot. You didn't know what to wear. You didn't know what to bring. You didn't know where to start. And you didn't even know enough to ask good questions. Some young fitness instructor at the gym was going to take one look at you, and scoff at your ignorance and lack of ability. Later, when the gym closed, you would likely be the hot topic of discussion over the water cooler.

It went even deeper, didn't it? Getting fit seemed daunting. After a lifetime of being sedentary, pumping iron seemed futile. How could you possibly go from YOUR body to THAT body? This is the time in life when you're expected to "slow down." Revving up your engines now seems like an obscene obsession with clinging to youth. And impossible to do.

And, as you've gotten older, you have begun to fear getting injured. You've discovered that the consequences of seemingly minor difficulties are magnified now, and recovery takes forever. Strength training has language like "buff," "ripped," and "cut." It's obviously going to be painful. You simply can't risk a strain, or even a sore muscle. Besides, you think you're pretty fragile. After all, you are . . . older.

Hit the nail right on the head, didn't we? Don't be surprised. Not only are many of our athletes older, but Jim Wharton himself is senior. We have a unique understanding of the heart and spirit of the older athlete.

So you can trust us when we say, "We know what you're going through. Now, get over it."

Don't be concerned about feeling foolish. Everybody starts at ground zero. Everybody in the gym had a first day. If they look like they know what they're doing now, it's only because they were willing to feel foolish for a moment. Believe us when we tell you that NO ONE will think you're an idiot. Get over being self-conscious. People at the gym are focused and self-absorbed in their own workouts. They aren't paying a bit of attention to you. And if they do notice you, they'll respect you. We promise. As for the instructors, they're trained to assist the beginner—and proud to do it. They aren't going to be laughing at you; they're going to be bragging about you.

As far as knowing what to wear and bring, we recommend setting an appointment at the gym, in advance of signing up. They'll be glad to give you an orientation session and a tour of the gym and all its facilities. You might even get a sample workout with an instructor who specializes in "first" encounters. Sneak a peek at what other people are wearing and pay attention to the bags in the locker room. You might notice towels, water bottles, stretch ropes, mats, sweat bands, lifting gloves, cosmetics, soap, shampoo, conditioner, razors, hair dryers, fresh clothing, plastic bags for wet things, radios, CD players, and tape players with headphones. Another way to decide what you need is to lay in the basics: a towel and a water bottle. Then, after your first session, decide if you need anything else. It's common for the "collection" to grow. We will tell you one little inside tip: brand-new stuff is a dead giveaway that you're a rookie. Well-worn clothing and a scuffed-up bag will make you less conspicuous.

Don't let your quest for fitness seem daunting. You aren't going to work out once and get fit. It's going to take time and work. Gains made in fitness are a lot like the losses in dieting. They happen one micron at a time. We have a friend who pranced into our clinic one day and announced happily, "My weight loss program is going great! Look at me! I've lost half a pound!" We knew she had been struggling with her weight for years, so we were effusive in our praise. "How long did it take you to lose the half a pound?" we inquired. "A month!" she cheered. We were confused by her enthusiasm. A month seemed a long time to us. Our confusion must have been evident. She explained simply, "I weigh less than I did a month ago. That was my TOP weight. I'll *never* be that heavy again. I'm on my way down to a normal weight. I'm making progress, don't you see?" Yes, we did. Her point was that ANY progress is still progress. The same is true with working out. You have to START! And whatever progress you make in your first day will put you ONE FULL DAY ahead of where you were yesterday. Yesterday, you were as unfit as you're ever going to be. *Ever.*

Don't worry about getting injured. If you're smart, you won't. FIRST, CLEAR YOUR PLANS WITH YOUR PHYSICIAN. In fact, you might even check in with a sports medicine physician. Then put your program together with realistic goals. Take it slowly. Remember that you're *always* in full control. (This is one of the great secret pleasures of working out!) Do what you want to and can do. If something hurts, knock it off. If you get tired, go home. But remember to come back. Fitness builds in increments that follow rest. You're far more likely to experience a breakthrough than a breakdown. And keep records so you can track your progress. It's a big boost to know that you can lift easily a weight that you couldn't budge a month before.

Being fit helps PREVENT injury. If you want to have the muscle integrity to stand tall, the skeletal integrity to avoid, slow, or slightly reverse osteoporosis, the flexibility to move easily and fluidly, and the stamina to keep moving, then you need to be fit. You deserve the benefits of glowing good health.

Our best advice is: GET MOVING! NOW!

> Whether I grow old or no,
> By the effect I do not know;
> But this I know, without being told,
> 'Tis time to live, if I grow old,
> 'Tis time short pleasures now to take,
> Of little life the best to make,
> And manage wisely the last stake.
>
> —Anacreon, 6th Century BC; Translated by
> Abraham Cowley (1618–1667)

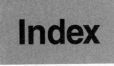

Index